Hearing, Taste and Smell

Hearing, Taste and Smell

Pathways of Perception

TORSTAR BOOKS
New York • Toronto

TORSTAR BOOKS INC.
41 Madison Avenue, Suite 2900
New York, NY 10010

THE HUMAN BODY
Hearing, Taste and Smell:
Pathways of Perception

Publisher
Bruce Marshall

Art Director
John Bigg

Editor
Jinny Johnson

Art Editor
David Fordham

Text Editor
Gwen Rigby

Researchers: Pip Morgan, Jazz Wilson

Director of Picture Research
Zilda Tandy

Picture Researchers: Mary Corcoran, Jessica Johnson, Sarah Marshall

Artists: Norman Barber, Mike Courtney, Frank Kennard, Michael Woods

Art Assistant: Carole McCleeve

Cover Design: Moonink Communications

Cover Art: Paul Giovanopoulos

Director of Production: Barry Baker

Production Coordinator: Janice Storr

Business Director: Candy Lee

Planning Assistant: Avril Essery

International Sales: Barbara Anderson

In conjunction with this series Torstar Books offers an electronic digital thermometer which provides accurate body temperature readings in large liquid crystal numbers within 60 seconds.

For more information write to:
Torstar Books Inc.
41 Madison Avenue, Suite 2900
New York, NY 10010

Authors

Philip Whitfield is a biologist and zoologist with a wide range of interests. He has written and contributed to many books, including *The Animal Family, Jungles, Rhythms of Life* and *The Biology of Parasitism* and has also published papers, including work on sensory systems, in many academic journals.

Mike Stoddart is a biologist and zoologist with particular interests in mammalian behavior and the study of olfaction. A foremost expert on smell, he has written many research papers on the subject and is the author of *The Ecology of Vertebrate Olfaction*. He has also contributed to many other books on the natural sciences including *The Animal Family, Jungles* and *Rhythms of Life*.

Biology and also serves as Chief of the Laboratory for Developmental Biology in the University's Gerontology Center. His research on the genetic basis of congenital defects of the head and neck has been widely published.

Lewis Thomas is Chancellor of the Memorial Sloan-Kettering Cancer Center in New York City and University Professor at the State University of New York, Stony Brook. A member of the National Academy of Sciences, Dr. Thomas has served on advisory councils of the National Institutes of Health. He has written *The Medusa and the Snail* and *Lives of a Cell*, which received the 1974 National Book Award in Arts and Letters.

Robert C. Blackmon is currently an Associate Professor of Audiology at California State University, Chico, where, in addition to teaching, he is the director of an audiology clinic. His research endeavors have been reported in numerous professional journals and texts, and he is frequently an invited speaker for professional as well as lay groups.

Gillian D. Sales is a lecturer in zoology at King's College, University of London. An expert in mammalian hearing abilities, she is author, with Professor J. P. Pye, of *Ultrasonic Communication by Animals*. She is at present engaged in research on ultrasonic communication and its role in the social biology of animals.

Series Consultants

Donald M. Engelman is Professor of Molecular Biophysics and Biochemistry and Professor of Biology at Yale. He has pioneered new methods for understanding cell membranes and ribosomes, and has also worked on the problem of atherosclerosis. He has published widely in professional and lay journals and lectured at many universities and international conferences. He is also involved with National Advisory Groups concerned with Molecular Biology, Cancer, and the operation of National Laboratory Facilities.

Stanley Joel Reiser is Professor of Humanities and Technology in Health Care at the University of Texas Health Science Center in Houston. He is the author of *Medicine and the Reign of Technology*; coeditor of *Ethics in Medicine: Historical Perspectives and Contemporary Concerns*; and coeditor of the anthology *The Machine at the Bedside*. He is the coeditor of the new International Journal of Technology Assessment in Health Care.

Harold C. Slavkin, Professor of Biochemistry at the University of Southern California, directs the Graduate Program in Craniofacial

Consultants for Hearing, Taste and Smell

Lloyd R. Dropkin is Assistant Professor of Otolaryngology at The New York Hospital–Cornell University Medical Center. He has specialized in this area of medicine throughout his career and is a member of the American Academy of Otolaryngology and a Fellow of the American College of Surgeons. He has published his research on the nasal cavity in professional journals.

Barry E. Hirsch is an Assistant Professor of Otolaryngology at Georgetown University Hospital, Washington, D.C. He is also a member of the attending staff at The Children's National Medical Center; The Washington Hospital Center; and the Veterans' Hospital. He has published numerous articles on infections and cancer of the head and neck.

Myra Engelman Lerch is an anthropologist who earned her M.A. degree in Speech Pathology and Audiology from California State University at Chico. Mrs. Lerch is currently Project Director for a series of workshops for parents of children with hearing impairment.

© **Torstar Books Inc. 1985**

**Library of Congress
Cataloging in Publication Data**

Whitfield, Philip.
    Hearing, taste, and smell.

    Includes index.
    1. Hearing. 2. Taste. 3. Smell. I. Stoddart,
D. Michael (David Michael) II. Title.
QP461.W476 1984   612'.86   84-8726

ISBN 0-920269-22-2 (The Human Body series)
ISBN 0-920269-29-X (Hearing, Taste and Smell)
ISBN 0-920269-30-3 (leatherbound)
ISBN 0-920269-31-1 (school ed.)

20 19 18 17 16 15 14 13 12 11
10   9   8   7   6   5   4   3   2

Printed in Belgium

Contents

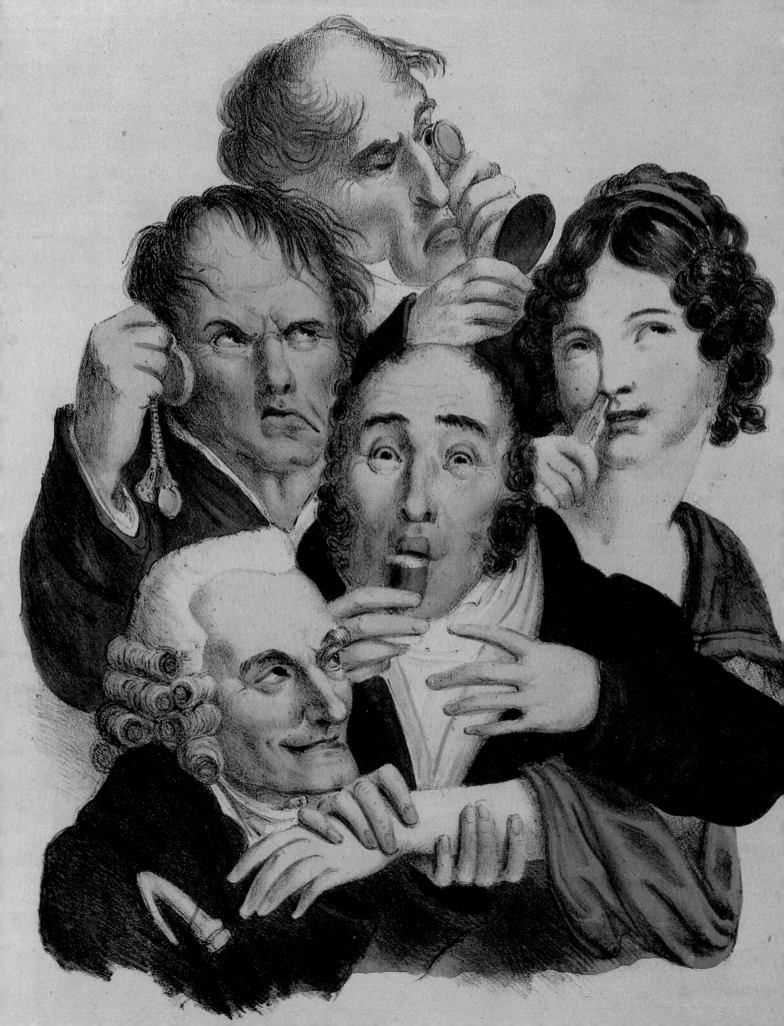

Introduction

The Alchemy of the Senses

In every waking moment, we are aware of the infinite complexity of the world around us. We are embedded in, and experience, a kaleidoscopic landscape. That landscape impinges on our conscious minds not as the staggering ferment itself, but as the filtered, modified and analogized version with which our senses provide us. Those sensory systems are at the same time the windows between the outer world and our consciousness and the walls that define the bounds of that inner world. There is a delicate balance between the vistas that the senses open up and the limits they set on our unaided sensibilities.

What is the hierarchical structure of our sensory abilities? Touch, temperature sense and pain seem the most generalized of these abilities, with apparatus for their reception all over the body surface. Vision, hearing, taste and smell, however, are all concentrated in the head. These four are the senses that connect us with other human beings and the rest of the world. In this series, *The Eye* revealed the wonders of human sight; this volume considers the remaining triumvirate: hearing, taste and smell.

The chemical senses, taste and smell, and the perception of sounds together provide almost boundless opportunities for human communication and for the sampling of the physical world around us. Through them physical things become sensations. For example, out there in the circumscribed world of physics, is a repetitive ripple of pressure changes in the air. The alchemy of ear, nerves and brain takes those waveforms and makes from them the experience of such melodic perfection as a Schubert quartet.

While finding out what science and medicine have to say concerning these three senses, it might be appropriate to remember the dualism—sound waves and Schubert. Whatever is known of the biochemistry, physiology, ultrastructure and genetics of these senses, human experience through them infinitely transcends such knowledge.

A humorous depiction of the five senses, published in 1823, shows these complex abilities at their most basic. In fact, as the following pages will reveal for three of the five, the senses link us to the world; they are our means of experiencing all that surrounds us and of communicating with others.

THE SATURDAY EVENING
POST

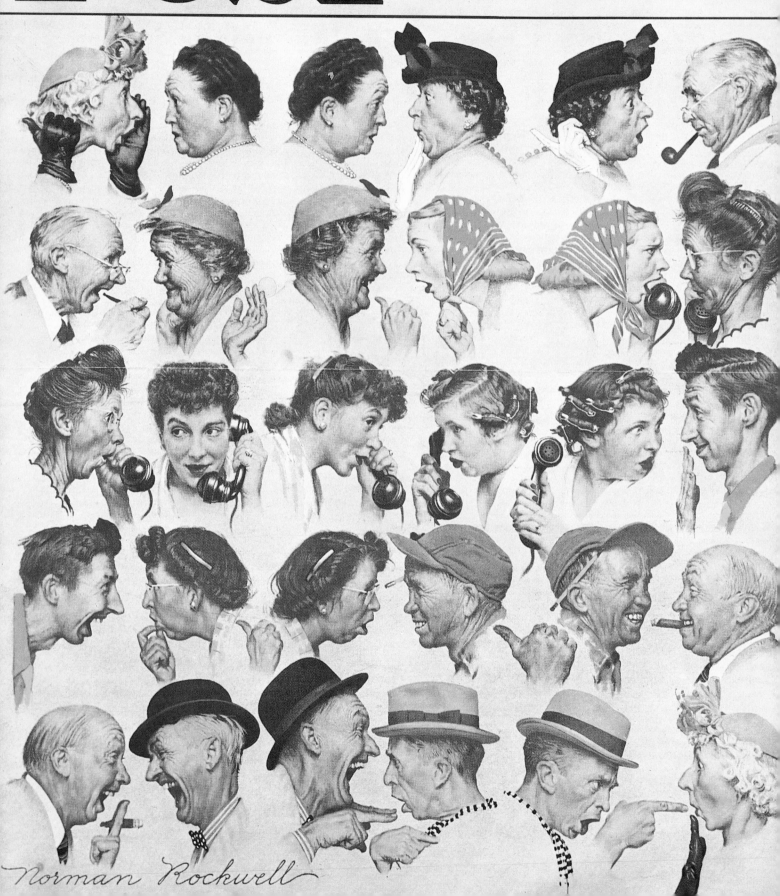

Norman Rockwell

Chapter 1

The Functioning of the Ear

"When I consider how my light is spent. . ." Thus Milton, the great seventeenth-century English poet, mused despairingly on the fact of his blindness, but he was apparently able to find stoical comfort in the thought that passivity had its own rewards: "They also serve who only stand and wait." Jonathan Swift struck perhaps a more realistic and bitter note concerning man's response to the loss of one of his senses when he wrote of his deafness:

> Deaf, giddy, helpless, left alone,
> To all my friends a burden grown.
> No more I hear the church's bell
> Then if it sang out for my knell;
> At thunder now no more I start
> Than at the rumbling of a cart. . . .

In six short, emotion-filled lines Swift describes the pathology, as well as the personal and social trauma, brought about by deafness. That the loss of hearing can so devastate a human being speaks powerfully for the central role that this sensory capacity plays in our lives. Speech is the magic thread that binds friends, families and societies together; it is the mode of communication that dramatically separates *Homo sapiens* from all other animals. That speech means so much to us is testimony to the extraordinary sensitivity and subtlety of the hearing system that interprets it.

Yet perceiving the speech of others is only one of the incredibly diverse functions of our ears. We can hear the softest footfall on a dark night, distinguish a baby's cry of pain from one of hunger or hear a single wrong note played by one instrument out of a hundred in a symphony orchestra. Because of their sense of hearing, piano tuners can earn a living, singers can have perfect pitch. In addition to these hearing skills, the ear is also the seat of less obvious senses related to gravity, body position and movement. Swift noted their disruption — giddiness — as well as the blank nothingness of the affliction of deafness.

In The Gossips, *painted in 1948 for the* Saturday Evening Post, *Norman Rockwell tells a humorous visual tale about the power of the spoken word. A piece of gossip is eagerly passed from ear to ear — no doubt undergoing subtle changes with each retelling — until it rebounds on its initiator. The expressions, ranging from horror to amusement, of those involved perfectly convey the flavor of the story under discussion.*

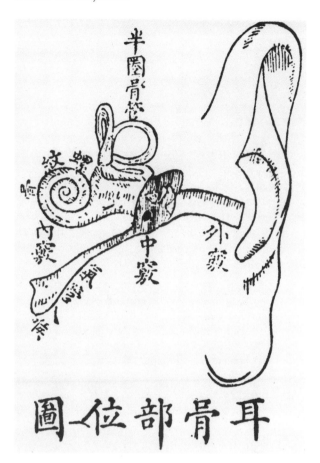

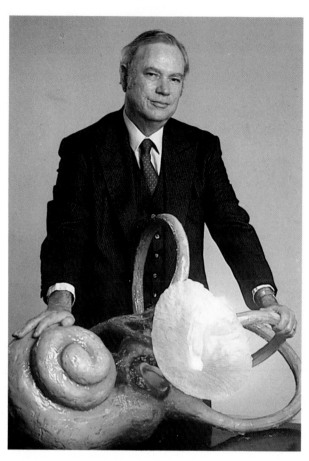

Knowledge of the sensitivities of the ears and the anatomical structures associated with them has accumulated unevenly through recorded history. Information was first systematized concerning the outer ear, then the middle ear and, lastly, the inner ear — an order related to one of increasing difficulties in observation. Let us pause briefly to look at the tripartite architecture of the ear. The outer ear is the obvious external portion, shaped like a cross between a squashed trumpet bell and a mollusk shell. It also comprises a tube, the external auditory meatus, which leads inward to the eardrum, or tympanum, which marks the boundary between the outer and the middle ear. The latter is an air-filled cavity, crossed by a chain of minute bones (the ossicles), which link up with parts of the inner ear. This inner ear consists of an intricate system of bony canals and membranous tubes, where the organs for hearing (the cochlea) and for the detection of gravity and movement are housed, buried inside bone.

The ancient Egyptians knew that the ear was associated with hearing. A papyrus, dating from about 1550 B.C., states: "For an ear that hears badly, use red lead and resin; grind to a powder, rub in fresh olive oil, frankincense and sea salt, syringe into the ear." Whether or not this concoction did much for the hard of hearing is open to question, but the instructions show that a detailed connection had been made between the ears and hearing. Because of the excellent opportunities for discovering details of human anatomy afforded by complex mummification rites, the Egyptians of this time, and probably earlier, discovered the Eustachian tube — the duct that leads from the middle ear to the nasopharynx. Given the times, it was a remarkable finding, but it generated a misunderstanding concerning the relationship

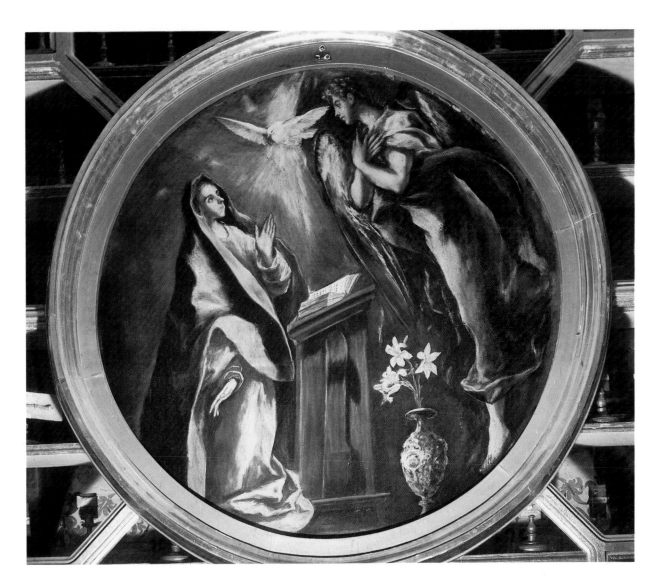

between the ears and breathing that persisted for over a millennium.

Naturally enough, the finding of an internal tube between nose and ear led to the suggestion that the ear was involved in respiration as well as hearing. The Egyptians surmised that "the breath of life passes by the right ear, the breath of death by the left ear." A thousand years later, Alcmaeon, a pupil of Pythagorus, was one of the earliest recorded Greek investigators and thinkers to be concerned with the functions of the ear. Around 580 B.C. he was describing (indeed rediscovering) the Eustachian tube and reiterating the Egyptian idea of a link between the ear and respiration. He stated that goats breathed through their ears. It was Hippocrates however, in about 460 B.C., who described the tympanic membrane, recognizing it as part of the organ of hearing, and Aristotle (384–322 B.C.), who first noted the coiled cochlea.

Most Romans scorned to soil their hands with the sordid practice of medicine — in their eyes a calling suited only to slaves and foreigners. They were, however, interested in knowledge relating to things medical. Of the great encyclopedia produced by Celsus (Aulus Cornelius) in the first century B.C., the eight books entitled *De Medicina* survive and demonstrate this interest. In Book VI, devoted to special subjects such as skin, eyes, teeth, venereal disease and the ears, are methods for shaking foreign bodies out of the ear canal and a recipe for an infusion for earache.

Galen, otherwise known as Claudius Galenus, a Greek born in Pergamum in Asia Minor, appears to have been the first to attempt a detailed explanation of the hearing function of the ear. He studied medicine at Alexandria and after, among other things, working as surgeon to a school for gladiators, he became surgeon to Marcus Aurelius

11

Andreas Vesalius (1514–64), the greatest anatomist of his time, numbered among his many achievements the first description of the malleus and the incus, two of the three bones of the middle ear.

The Eustachian tube, the passage that connects the throat and ear, is named after sixteenth-century Italian anatomist, Bartolommeo Eustachio, who first fully described this tube and its function.

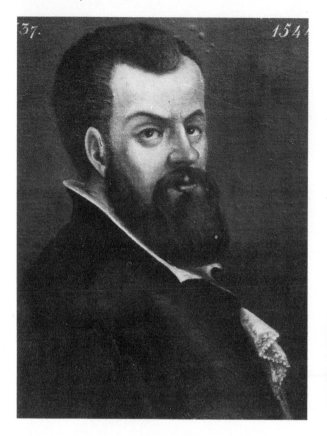

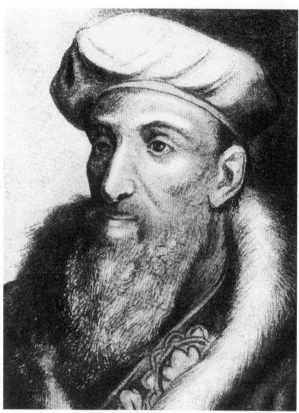

in Rome. By his dissections of many animals — particularly dogs, pigs and apes — Galen found that the ear was connected to the brain by the auditory nerve. He realized that the outer ear functioned as a collector of sounds and was, as he put it, "especially tuned to the sounds of the human voice." He also provided a worthwhile description of the gross structure of the inner ear and was the first to call this maze of bony membranous passages "the labyrinth," a term we still use.

The breakthrough in the understanding of the ear's function constituted by Galen's discoveries was not fully capitalized on until the Renaissance. A sudden flowering in anatomical studies in the great universities of Italy at this time provided much new knowledge on the structure of and relationships between the middle and inner ear. Andreas Vesalius (1514–64) was, without question, the foremost anatomist of the Renaissance period, and he reformed the study of human anatomy with

the publication of his *De Humani Corporis Fabrica* in 1543. Appointed to the Chair of Anatomy at Padua in his twenties, Vesalius was the first investigator to provide an accurate description of the first two bones of the middle ear ossicle chain, the malleus and the incus. The innermost of these tiny, yet so important, bones, the stapes, was described a few years later by Gian Filippo Ingrassia, an Italian scientist at the University of Naples. Vesalius also described the eardrum in some detail as well as the two membranous "windows," which connect the middle ear with the seat of the sensation of hearing, the cochlea. A remarkable and productive scientist, Andreas Vesalius died after being shipwrecked during a pilgrimage to visit the Holy Sepulcher in Jerusalem.

One other Renaissance scholar must be mentioned before we jump forward 400 years to our present understanding of the senses that reside in the ear. Bartolommeo Eustachio (1520–74) held the Chair of Anatomy in Rome and, in 1562, published

Epistola de Auditus Organis, his treatise on the ear. Although this work was almost unknown until the eighteenth century, it has a strong claim to being the earliest to deal exclusively with the ear. Fitting, then, that the name of Eustachio lives on, tied irrevocably to the tube that he first fully described, even though the Egyptians and Greeks knew of its existence long before.

These men were the builders who laid the first, all-important stones in the edifice of our understanding of the ear and its functions. The intellectual construction is now much more complex than Renaissance minds could have dreamed. Yet it is probably not fanciful to imagine that a time-transported Vesalius or Eustachio would soon feel at ease with the molecular biologists, electron microscopists and neurophysiologists, who today grapple with the mysteries of the ear. Shared scientific curiosity would bridge the centuries.

The Nature of Sound

To comprehend how the human ear, indeed the ear of any animal, perceives sound, the nature of sound itself must first be understood. Sound is a method of energy transfer. Although sound originates from the motion, or vibration, of an object, it is not the actual vibration of that object that we normally hear but the effect of that vibration. The vibrating object might be a ringing bell, a vibrant violin or a person's vocal cords. The movements cause disturbances in the air, and it is these disturbances which travel to our ears and are then experienced as sound. Human hearing has evolved to operate in air and it is in air that most hearing occurs, but sound travels through a wide variety of mediums and thus can also be transmitted well through most compact solids and water. We can perceive sounds underwater by the vibrations transmitted to the cochlea via the bones of the skull, but sound cannot travel through a vacuum. The sound of a ringing alarm clock inside a vacuum chamber dies away to nothing as the air inside the chamber is removed.

Still air consists of molecules of nitrogen, oxygen and carbon dioxide, which are in constant random motion. Imagine the diaphragm of an audio loudspeaker beginning to vibrate in such air; the in-and-out movements of the diaphragm are transmitted to

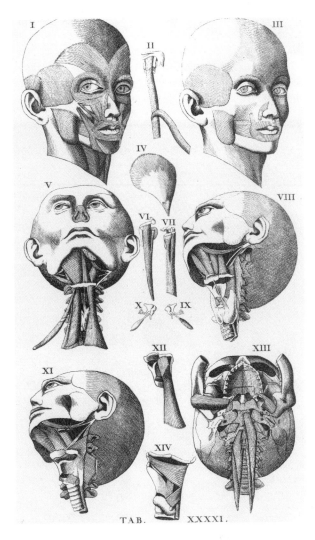

TAB. XXXXI.

the closely adjacent air molecules, which are forced to move in the same direction as the diaphragm. As the diaphragm moves outward, the nearby molecules are displaced from their average resting positions, and they, in turn, pass this movement onto molecules close to them in a kind of chain reaction. When the diaphragm moves back in the opposite direction, the displacements occur in the opposite direction. The balanced nature of these events means that individual molecules do not change their resting position. There is no overall mass movement of air as sound passes through it; instead the disturbance passes outward by a form of molecular "shunting." A helpful analogy might be to think of a line of railroad cars hitched together. If a locomotive rams into one end of the line, a machine-gun rattle of colliding bumpers will run rapidly from one end of the line to the other, although no individual car will move more than a few inches. In the same way, a sound disturbance passes rapidly through air, while the individual

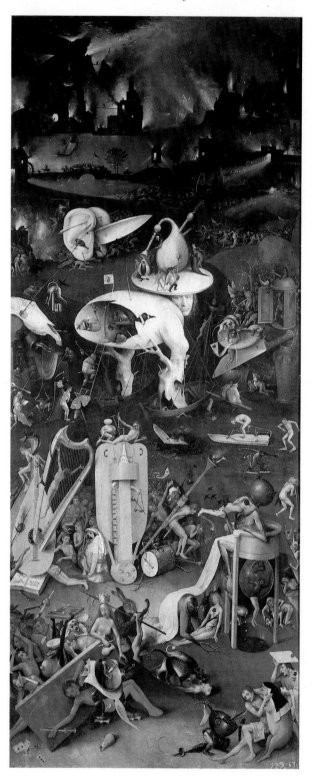

molecules transmitting it make only small movements from their resting positions.

For the duration of a sound disturbance in air, the air molecules move alternately closer together than normal and then farther apart than normal. The first phase of activity represents an area of compression of the air, the second an area of lowered pressure, or rarefaction. Sound, then, is transmitted as a series of oscillating displacements of air molecules, which give rise to waves of compression and rarefaction, spreading ever outward from the sound-emitting object. These sound waves can be thought of in a number of related ways. On a graph, a plot against time of the displacements of air molecules from their resting positions during the passage of a sound has the shape of a regular, or sine, wave. A similar sinusoidal waveform is generated if one considers the oscillating pressure changes (the compressions and rarefactions) of sound through time. This same regularly alternating form is obtained by reference to the changing degrees of either air displacement or pressure at one instant as sound travels through a region of air-filled space.

High and Low Frequencies

The technical terms used to describe waveforms of this type have great practical significance when discussing the physical characteristics of sound and hearing. For example, the repeat duration of the wave in time (from peak to peak) is called the wave's period. The period is reciprocally related to the wave's frequency, which is the number of cycles of a sound wave that passes a given point in one second—the shorter the period, the greater the frequency and vice versa.

Here is a topic specifically relevant to human perception of sound, for the sensation we describe as the pitch of a sound is directly related to its frequency. High notes have high frequencies and low notes, low. Technically, a frequency of one cycle per second (1 cps) is a frequency of one Hertz, or Hz. Most human beings can perceive a range of sound frequencies between about 20 Hz (20 cps) and 20,000 Hz (20,000 cps). The former sound is an extremely low note, felt more as a vibration than a sound, while the latter is a high-pitched, thin whine.

14

Sound is a mode of energy transfer through air or other substances. The composite diagram shows how undisturbed molecules of air — represented as motionless pendulums — are set in motion by a vibrating membrane such as a loudspeaker. As the molecules oscillate about their resting position, they are compressed, or rarefied, as the sound waves pass. Patterns resembling real wave forms (bottom diagram) are produced by drawing out graphs of the two types of characteristic that change with time at a point in space: the amplitude of the displacement which the air molecules undergo, and the pressure changes in air.

In air and at room temperature, sound travels at about 370 yards per second. Given this fact, the frequency of a sound wave can be related to the actual wavelength, that is, the distance between two adjacent points of maximum air compression. The wavelength equals the velocity of the sound divided by its frequency, so a low note (20 Hz) has a wavelength of 56 feet. In other words, the compression peaks in the air are some 56 feet apart. The highest note we can hear without artificial aids (20,000 Hz) has a wavelength of only 0.67 inches. This means that the compressions hitting the eardrum are less than three-quarters of an inch apart.

The wavelength of a sound determines the way in which that sound behaves when it encounters an object in its path and so it is important in many aspects of the reception of sound waves by human and other animal ears. Sounds are reflected by objects with dimensions bigger than those of the sound's wavelength, but they pass more or less unimpeded around objects smaller than the wavelength. When sounds encounter obstacles with dimensions about equal to their own wavelength, they are scattered in all directions. Such considerations affect the way in which, for example, the pinna interacts with sounds of different frequency. And, in the world of animal sound communication, they also mean that low notes, that is, long wavelength sounds, are ideal for sound signaling in places where such objects as tree trunks stand between the calling animal and the listening animal. Where sounds must be efficiently reflected back along their previous paths — the echolocation "radar" signals of bats for instance — extremely high-frequency sounds are used.

Bats use sounds way above the human hearing range, with frequencies up to 200,000 Hz (ultrasonic sound). The wavelength of such a sound is about 1.5 millimeters and will bounce off even a small moth, since the wavelength is smaller than the target's dimensions.

Analyzing Complex Sounds

The smooth, simple waveforms of pure notes are found only rarely in the sound environment of human beings. Ordinary noises, particularly the sounds of human speech, are made up of complex

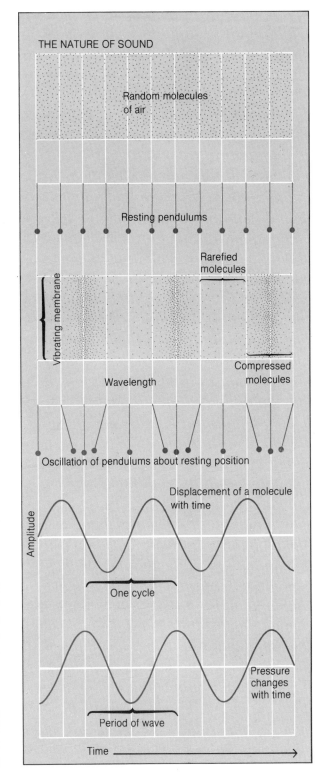

THE NATURE OF SOUND

Random molecules of air

Resting pendulums

Vibrating membrane

Rarefied molecules

Wavelength

Compressed molecules

Oscillation of pendulums about resting position

Amplitude

Displacement of a molecule with time

One cycle

Period of wave

Pressure changes with time

Time

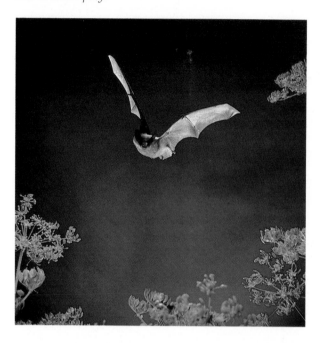

mixtures of frequency patterns. When tones are added together in this way, new, complicated waveforms are generated, which depend on the tones being mixed and on the time relationships between them. In his famous theorem, the French scientist, J. B. J. Fourier, showed that all repetitive waveforms, no matter how complicated, can be considered to be a mixture of simple sine waves. The disentangling of these simple components of the complex whole is called a Fourier analysis. Such analyses are important in many scientific contexts, when complex waves of all types are examined, but, without our giving any conscious thought to it, our ears do the same trick. The ear analyzes complex sounds into their constituent parts and so performs a Fourier analysis.

The loudness of a sound together with its pitch, as defined above, are probably its two most important characteristics from an animal's point of view; but what are we actually describing when one sound is said to be loud, another soft? Loudness refers to the perceived intensity of a sound wave, and it is directly related to the rate at which a sound is transferring energy. The intensity, or loudness, of a sound at a particular distance from the vibrating object producing it is the rate of energy transfer per second (that is, its power) as measured by the

sound per unit area. As we have said, the energy transfer is carried out by the vibrations of air molecules.

The quietest sound audible to the human ear operating at maximum efficiency has an intensity of about 0.000000000001 watt per square meter. To take an example near the other end of the spectrum of sound loudness, the noise of a Boeing 707, fully loaded and taking off from an airport, can be 10 watts per square meter. It is one of the loudest noises we hear and is about ten thousand billion times as powerful as the quietest sound that we can perceive. This huge range of loudness sensitivity shows the impressive flexibility of the human organs of hearing. It is also the central rationale for the internationally accepted measurement system for sound intensity.

Because such a wide variation in sound intensity falls within our sensitivity range, any linear scale of measurement rapidly becomes cumbersome. On a linear scale, the quietest whisper would be, perhaps, equal to one intensity unit, while a jet engine would have an intensity of 10,000,000,000,000 units (ten trillion). If reports on environmental impacts of airport noise pollution had to be written using units of that type, they would be dominated by strings of zeros. In an attempt to solve this practical problem, a nonlinear scale is normally used to measure intensity. A reference intensity, usually 10 watts per square meter, is used as the basis of this system, which works on the concept of ratios. Each tenfold increase in sound intensity over the reference level is called a Bel, in honor of Alexander Graham Bell one inventor of the telephone. On this scale, the jet engine, 10^{13} times louder than the reference intensity, would have an intensity of 13 Bels. Because a Bel is a rather large increase, tenths of a Bel, or decibels (dB), are used as the standard unit in practice. Using the decibel scale, the jet engine would have an intensity of 13×10, or 130 decibels.

Due to its basis in logarithmic ratios, the way in which the decibel scale behaves when intensity changes is often counterintuitive. If 6 volts are needed to run a radio, the desired power can be obtained by using two 3 volt batteries. Decibel intensities do not behave in this commonsense way. A noise of 90 decibels together with another of 90 decibels do not give 180 decibels. This is because

Pictures taken by a scanning electron microscope enable us to look at the three-dimensional structure of biological material. These nerve fibers in the organ of Corti, are seen at hundreds of times actual size.

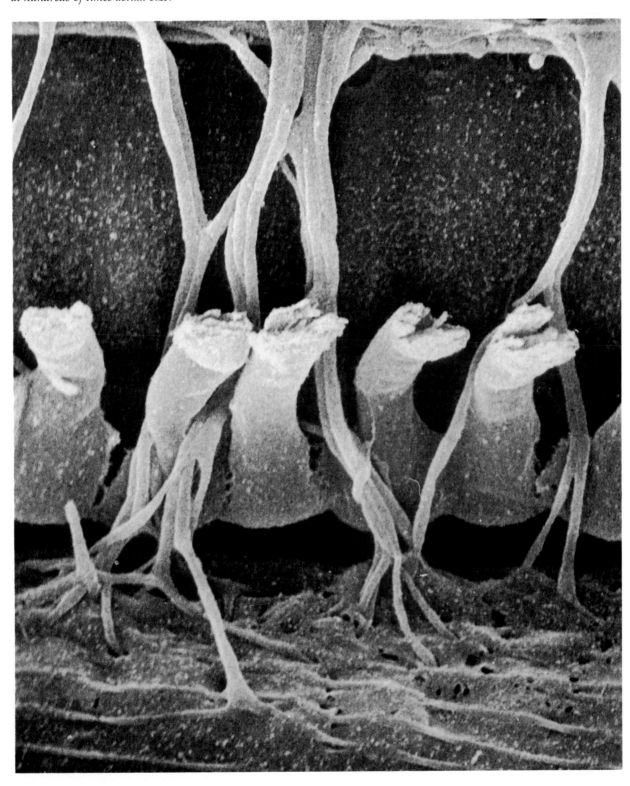

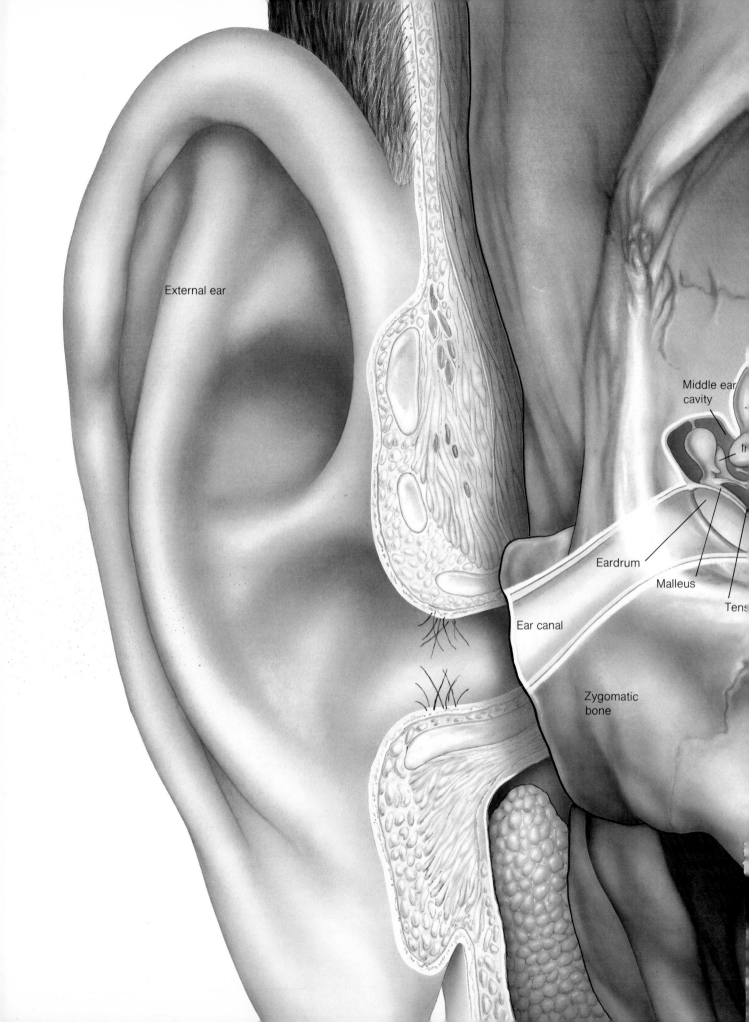

External ear

Middle ear
cavity

In

Eardrum

Malleus

Tens

Ear canal

Zygomatic
bone

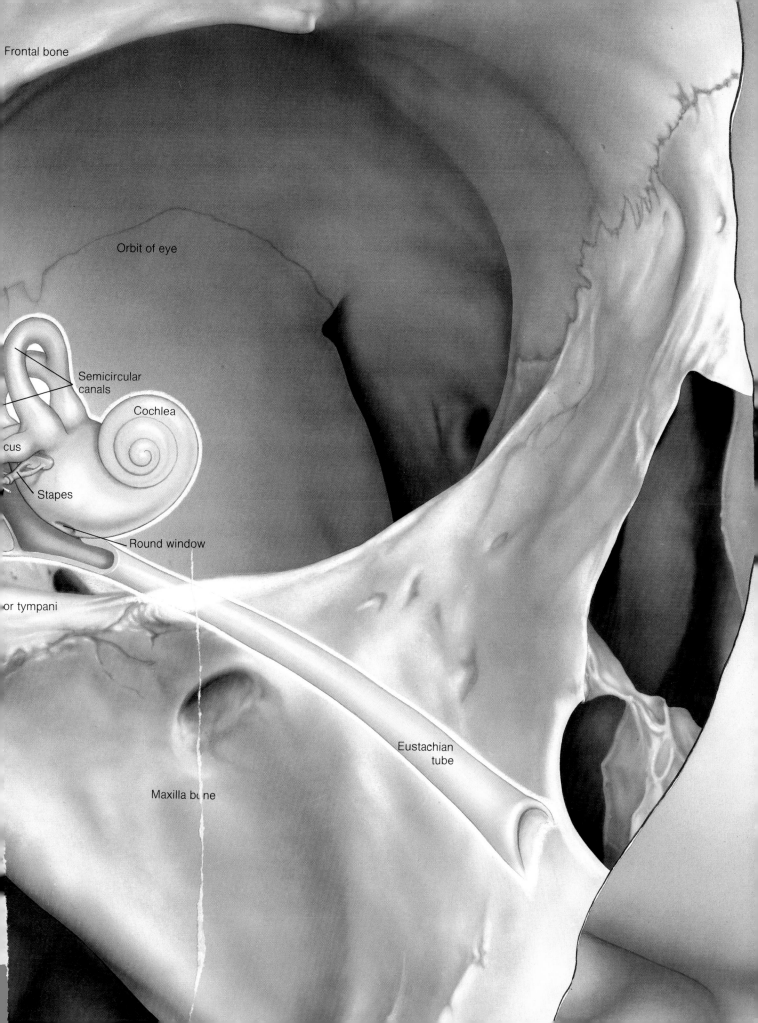

Frontal bone

Orbit of eye

Semicircular
canals

Cochlea

cus

Stapes

Round window

or tympani

Eustachian
tube

Maxilla bone

ACOUSTIQUE.

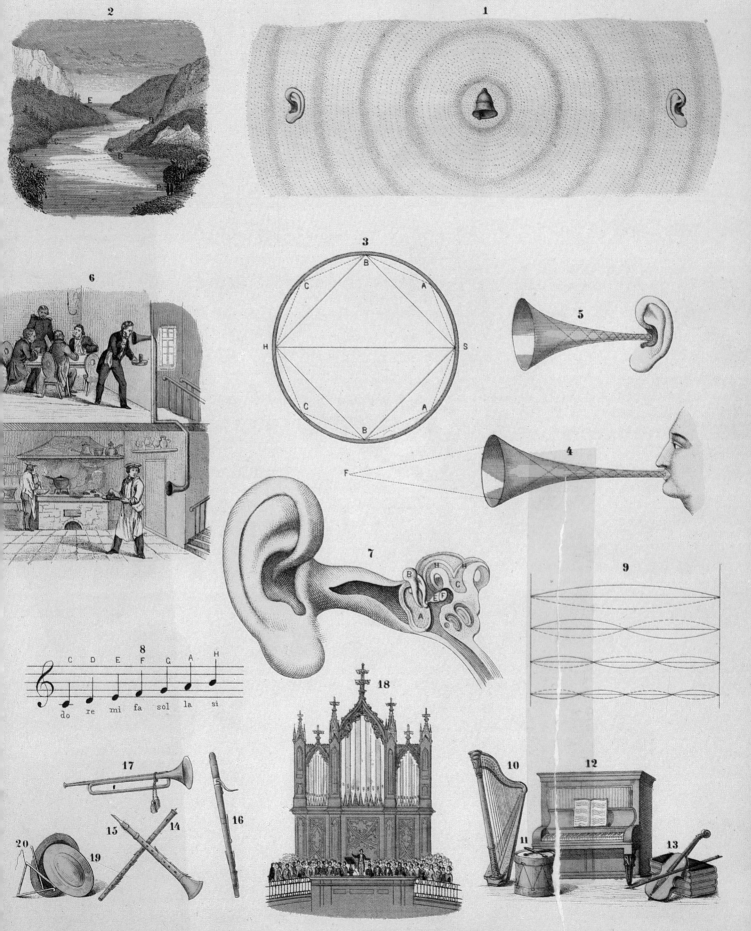

A plate from J. T. Desagulier's Mathematical Elements of Natural Philosophy, *published in 1747, shows equipment used in experiments to test levels of sound in different air pressure.*

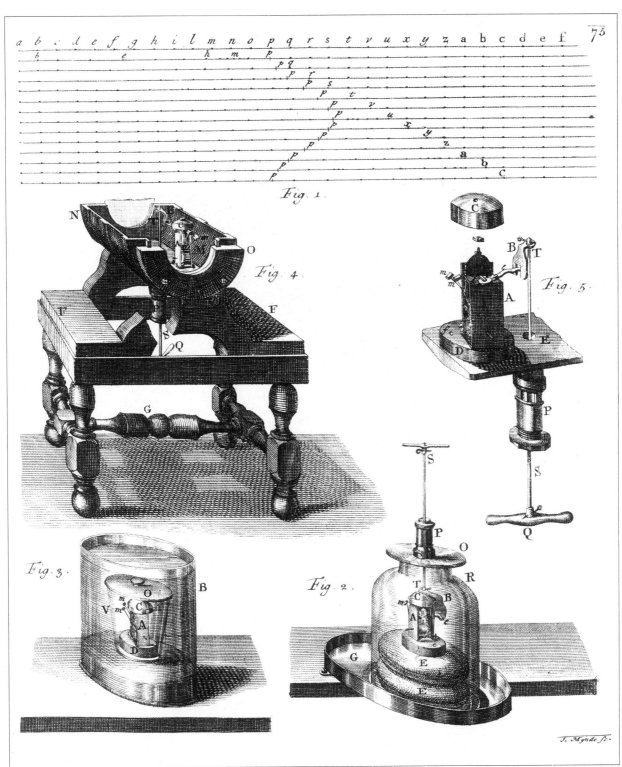

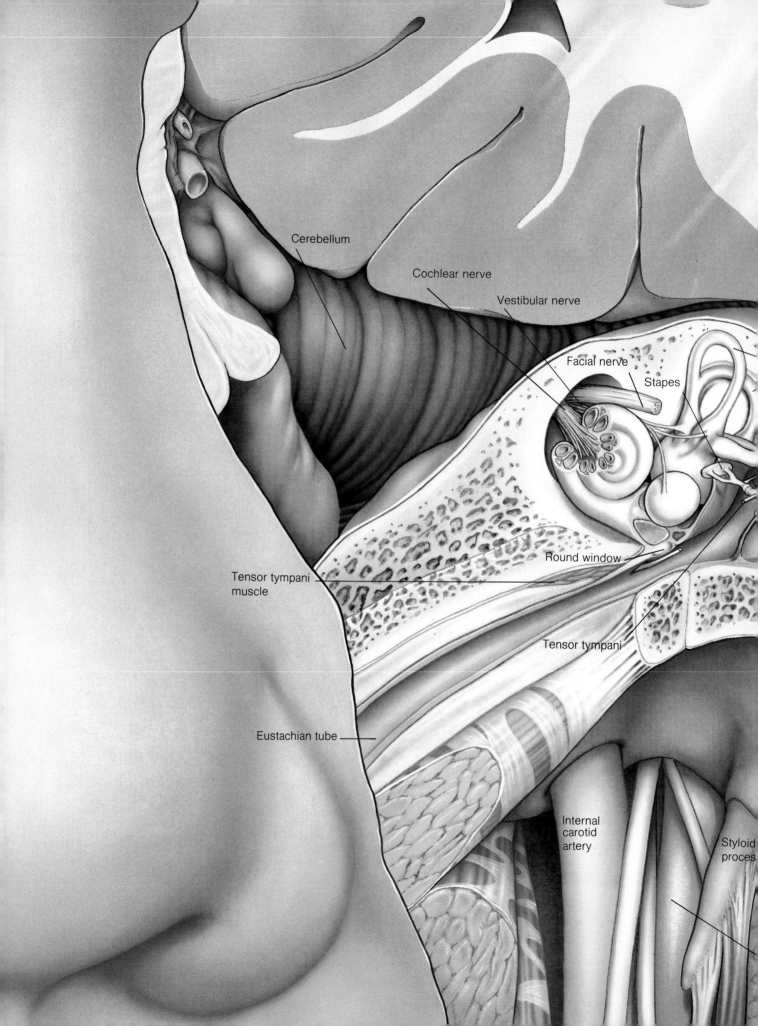

Cerebellum

Cochlear nerve

Vestibular nerve

Facial nerve

Stapes

Round window

Tensor tympani
muscle

Tensor tympani

Eustachian tube

Internal
carotid
artery

Styloid
proces

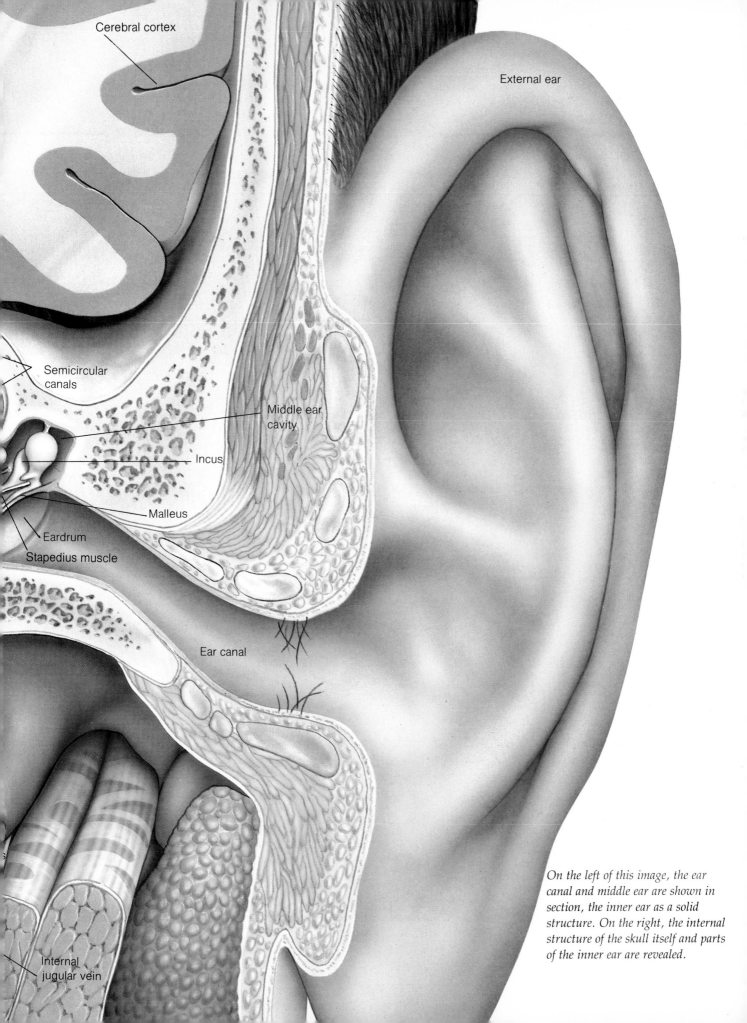

Cerebral cortex

External ear

Semicircular
canals

Middle ear
cavity

Incus

Malleus

Eardrum

Stapedius muscle

Ear canal

internal
jugular vein

*On the left of this image, the ear
canal and middle ear are shown in
section, the inner ear as a solid
structure. On the right, the internal
structure of the skull itself and parts
of the inner ear are revealed.*

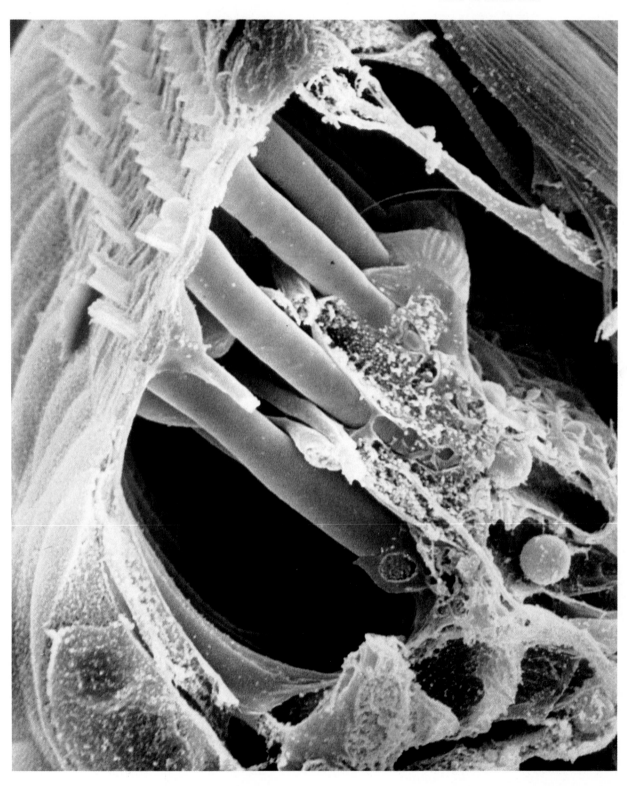

A scanning electron micrograph of part of the organ of Corti in the inner ear reveals the three-dimensional structure of this complex organ at many hundreds of times its actual size.

in logarithms, when a value is doubled, the logarithm value is not multiplied by two, but the logarithm of 2 is added to the original value. If a sound intensity is doubled, it increases by the logarithm of 2, which is 0.3. Thus the sound increases by 0.3 Bels, or 3 decibels. In the strange world of sound intensity measurement, 90 decibels plus 90 decibels equals 93 decibels. Whenever a sound intensity doubles, an increase of 3 decibels —more precisely of 3.0103 decibels—is obtained.

Decreasing Loudness

One final aspect of the physics of sound needs mention before we begin a more detailed scrutiny of the means by which our ears trap and analyze sound waves. This concerns the way in which the loudness of a sound decreases with increasing distance from the emitter of the sound energy. Two factors operate to bring about the apparently obvious conclusion that the farther away we are from, for example, people shouting, the quieter they sound. Straightforward enough, but why does it always happen?

The first part of the answer is connected with the way a sound spreads out from the vibrating object. If not impeded, sound spreads equally in all directions, and, at any instant, the outer moving surface of sound-disturbed air is sphere-shaped. As we get farther and farther from the source, the sphere gets bigger and bigger, and, as the wave front expands, the energy is spread over an increasingly greater area. All the energy that passes through a certain area at a fixed distance from the sound source in a specific interval of time will pass through an area four times as big in this time if the distance from the source is doubled. Intensity, therefore, decreases with distance owing to "energy spreading." Technically, it decreases with the inverse of the distance squared—a rapid decline rate.

The second reason for the decrease of loudness with distance is a rather surprising one. Sound exhausts itself by heating the air, and, as a sound wave passes through a volume of air, not all of the energy emitted by the sound source reaches the outer edge of the volume. Some of it is "lost" in warming the air it passes through. Such heat losses are proportionately greater for high-frequency, short wavelength sound than for low-frequency,

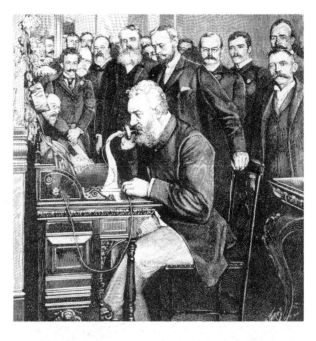

long wavelength sound. This means that, for efficient communication by animals over long distances, low notes are far more effective than high notes are.

The Functioning of the Human Ear

To reiterate, the ear divides conveniently into three interconnected compartments — the outer, middle and inner ears. The division is helpful, since it enables the extraordinarily complex activities of the ear to be described in manageable and reasonably distinct sections. The three regions of the ear are separated in a clear-cut way because, as well as being derived from absolutely disparate embryological origins, they are also exquisitely specialized for their own roles in the sequence of events from sound vibrations in the air to the sensation of sound in the consciousness.

The outer ear, consisting of the pinna and the external ear canal, performs various important functions. In particular, these regions of the ear modify the nature of the sounds reaching the eardrum in order to increase the sensitivity of the whole system to the particular sound frequencies that are crucial in the analysis of human speech. They also enable us to pinpoint the direction from which a sound comes. How are these desirable

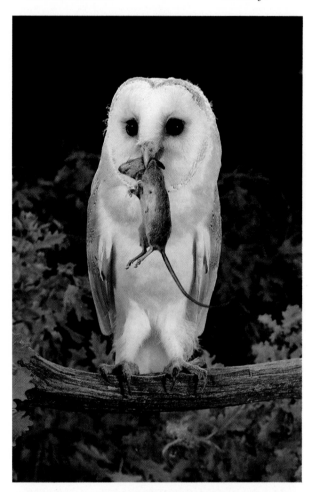

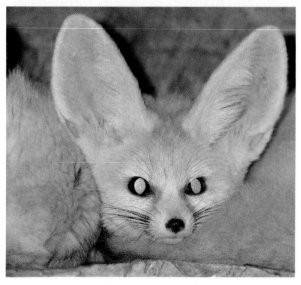

abilities built into the organization of the outer ear?

Many important speech characteristics exist in the frequency range between 2000 and 5000 Hz. It is precisely in this range that the shapes and dimensions of the pinna and ear canal produce a "gain" in the efficiency of sound transfer from the outside world to the eardrum. The gain is the result of a "tuning" of these spaces. The bowl-shaped structure, the concha, which leads into the canal, resonates at 5000 Hz, whereas the canal resonates at about 2500 Hz. In this way, the outer ear operates as a specific amplifier of the frequencies of human speech. Even before it impinges on the eardrum, a sound has been usefully manipulated by the spaces through which it is forced to pass.

Localizing Sounds

As animals go, man is a hopeless localizer of sounds. A fennec fox listening for termites in the ground beneath it, a barn owl pouncing with deadly precision on a mouse in complete darkness or a bat swooping on a tiny moth would all consider us to be handicapped in this capacity. One of our problems is that we cannot move our sound-gathering antennae, the pinnae, to home in on a sound. Watch a cat move its ears to point backward or forward in a fraction of a second and compare that controlled flexibility with the stolid immobility of our own ears. Despite this relative inadequacy, humans are still able to localize a sound to positions left or right, front or back, above or below the head.

Intensity and timing differences in the sound waves striking the two ears are the most important cues for human sound localization. The left-right sensitivity is explained by the fact that sound coming from the right-hand side will meet the right ear before the left and be more intense at the right ear — recollect the previous explanation of intensity decline with distance. Up-down and front-back sensitivities cannot, however, depend on such differences because, in all those instances, the sound reaches the two ears at the same time and with approximately the same intensity. The localization information comes from the effects of the concha and the pinna itself.

When a sound comes from behind the ear, the directly transmitted sound wave interferes with the wave scattered off the edge of the pinna, reducing

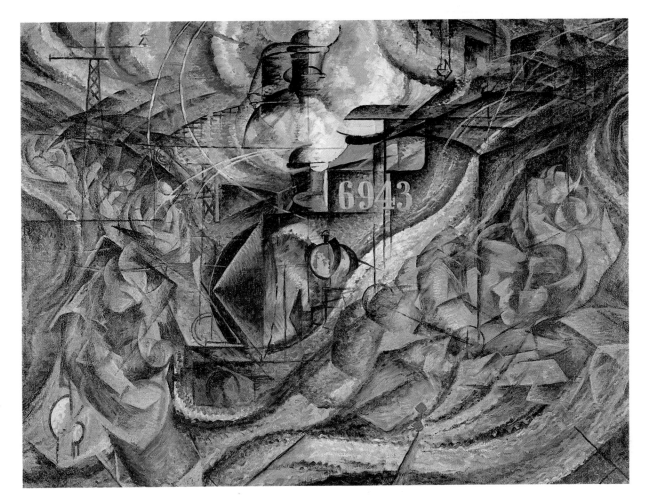

the intensity of the frequencies in the range 3000 to 6000 Hz reaching the eardrum. As the source of the sound moves around to the front of the head, these interference effects subside, and the relevant intensities increase proportionately. Front-to-rear sound localization probably depends on subtle, unconscious assessments of these relationships between frequency and intensity. Similar types of change in frequency spectra are used for judgments about the height of a sound source.

The Functions of the Middle Ear

The middle ear acts as a crucial intermediary in the processing of sound energy. Situated between the outer ear, which collects and channels the sound, and the inner ear, where the essential receptor cells are positioned, the middle ear structures link these two zones of the ear with exquisite and controlled efficiency.

An air-filled cavity, the middle ear is bounded on the outer side by the eardrum, or tympanic membrane, which functions as an airtight seal between outer and middle ears. The Eustachian tube, a narrow channel about one and a half inches long, connects the middle ear directly with the outside world. From its opening in the pharyngeal portion of the nose, this tube travels upward, backward and to the side to enter the floor of the middle ear. The smallest bones in the human body, the auditory ossicles cross the cavity of the middle ear. These bones, the malleus, incus and stapes, form a linked chain, joined at one end to the inner surface of the eardrum and at the other to a membranous partition, the oval window, which adjoins the fluid

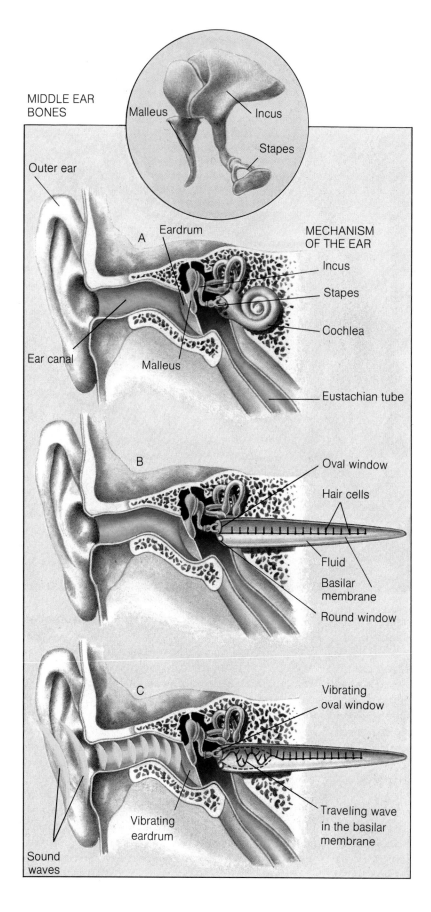

MIDDLE EAR
BONES

Malleus · Incus

Stapes

Outer ear

A · Eardrum

MECHANISM
OF THE EAR

Incus

Stapes

Cochlea

Ear canal

Malleus

Eustachian tube

B

Oval window

Hair cells

Fluid

Basilar
membrane

Round window

C

Vibrating
oval window

Vibrating
eardrum

Traveling wave
in the basilar
membrane

Sound
waves

A visualization of sound waves from a nineteenth-century book, Natural Philosophy, *shows the condensed waves formed when a clapper hits a bell and the rarefied waves during the periods of silence between its ringing* (right).

In 1826, two gentlemen set up an experiment on Lake Geneva to try and assess the speed of sound in water (right). *The receiver of the signals is here shown with his extraordinary underwater ear trumpet. Sound does, in fact, travel more quickly through water than through air of the same temperature. The warmer the water (or air), the faster the sound travels.*

The auditory apparatus for turning sound waves into mechanical vibrations is shown schematically in this series of images. The inset shows the linked bones of the middle ear: the malleus, incus and stapes. (A) These tiny bones fit into the middle ear cavity with the malleus attached to the eardrum and the stapes footplate to the oval window at the base of the cochlea. (B) For the sake of clarity, the diagram shows a straightened-out cochlea, with the hair cell receptors protruding from the basilar membrane. (C) When sound waves impinge on the eardrum, vibrations pass from there through the middle ear bones to the inner ear. A traveling wave is set up in the basilar membrane, which stimulates a subpopulation of hair cells that send impulses to the brain.

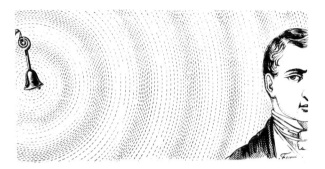

From a nineteenth-century work on sound, this experiment shows that sound needs a medium in which to travel. The plunger operates a bell, but its ringing is only heard when there is air in the jar.

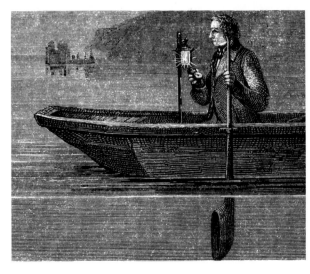

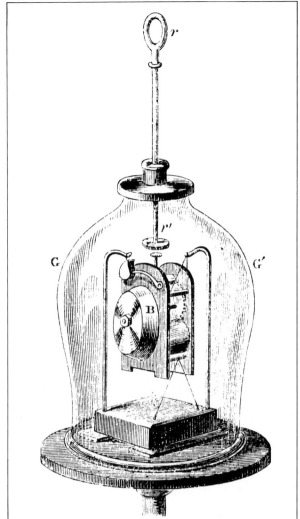

contents of the inner ear. Although the ossicles are spoken of as lying in the cavity of the middle ear, bones cannot actually be in unprotected contact with the air anywhere in the body. The ossicles, and the muscles and ligaments connected to them, are actually suspended in the cavity and "wrapped" in extensions of the living wall of the chamber.

The function of the middle ear is to transform variations in air pressure in the ear canal (produced by incoming sound waves) into equivalent pressure variations in the fluids of the inner ear. This transformation is required because, as we shall see, the receptors in the inner ear are stimulated by these fluid pressure alterations. The task of the middle ear, then, is to transform vibrations in air into vibrations in liquid.

Such transference is intrinsically difficult to produce. If sound waves impinge directly on a liquid surface, some 99.9 percent of the sound energy is reflected away from the liquid without affecting it in any way. Only a tiny fraction of the sound energy enters the liquid. If one were to remove the middle ear so that the round window of the inner ear took the place of the eardrum, the incoming sound waves would be unable to stimulate the inner ear fluids directly. In technical terms, this hypothetical piece of organic engineering would be inadequate because of an "impedance mismatch" between the air of the ear canal and the liquids of the inner ear. What is required of the middle ear is that it should overcome the impedance problem by increasing the air pressure changes in the outer ear into much greater pressures concentrated on the oval window.

The eardrum, ossicle chain and oval window constitute a system which achieves this pressure enhancement by two independent mechanisms that operate ·simultaneously when sounds are heard. One mechanism relates to the way in which

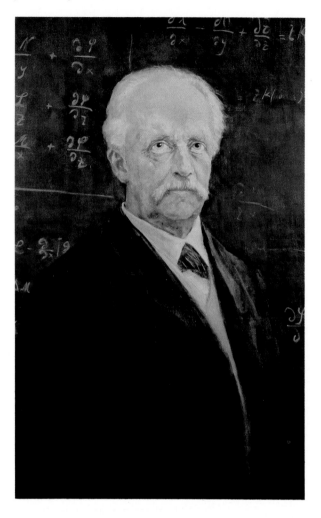

the ossicles act as levers, the other to the surface areas of the eardrum and the oval window. The linked series of events that takes a sound from the ear canal to the inner ear shows us how the mechanisms operate.

Sounds in the ear canal cause the eardrum to vibrate with complex patterns. First demonstrated by Helmholtz in 1868, the patterns of the vibrations vary with the sound frequency. Their complexity is largely due to the complicated structure of the eardrum, which has a stiff rim and a concave outer surface; it is set obliquely in the canal and is divided into relatively floppy and relatively taut regions. The complex patterns of vibration apparently allow extremely efficient transfer of acoustic energy, in frequencies below 10,000 Hz, from canal to middle ear. For frequencies over 10,000 Hz, this energy transfer becomes increasingly less efficient.

Because the "handle" of the malleus is attached along one inner radius of the eardrum, the vibrations directly activate the ossicle chain. Links between the three bones, and fibrous attachments between the bones and the wall of the middle ear cavity, ensure that rocking movements of the malleus — caused by eardrum vibrations — are themselves passed onto the innermost ossicle, the stapes. In fact, the geometry of the ossicle chain is such that it amplifies the mechanical forces applied by the stapes on the oval window. A force at the malleus end of the chain has been increased by about a third by the time it reaches the stapes end.

A much greater amplification of pressure level is achieved by the second mechanism, which is related to input and output area ratios. The eardrum is oval in shape, with a maximum diameter of about 10 millimeters and a minimum of 8 to 9 millimeters. Its effective vibrating area is about 55 square millimeters. The so-called footplate of the stapes, the bone plunger that activates the inner ear, has an area of only about 3.2 square millimeters. The force per unit area at the footplate is, therefore, massively increased because this force — already boosted by about 30 percent in the ossicle chain — is being applied over a considerably reduced area. An analogy may help to clarify this point. A woman standing on a cork tile floor with sneakers on her feet makes no impression on the floor covering. The same woman wearing stiletto-heeled shoes makes dimples in the floor. With the second pair of shoes on, she is applying the same force to the floor but over a much-reduced area. The force per unit area of floor is greatly increased, and the effect on the floor is greater.

This second amplification factor in the middle ear is the ratio of the two areas involved, that is, 55 to 3.2 or about seventeen times. Including the effect of the ossicle lever, the total middle-ear-induced amplification of incoming energy is about twenty-two times. This tremendous multiplication of force levels overcomes the impedance mismatch between air and fluid mentioned above.

The middle ear, though, has more sophisticated functions than simply that of a chamber containing a "coupling-rod" of bones. To start off with, the

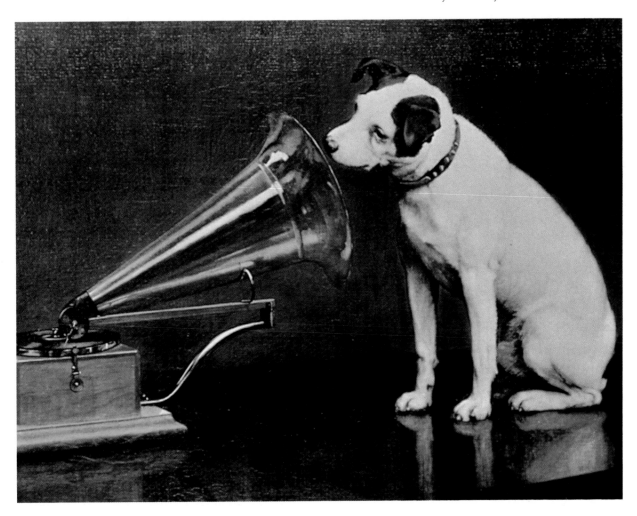

patterned vibrations of the eardrum depend on air pressures on each side of this airtight membrane being equal. If they were not, the eardrum would bulge inward or outward, depending on the direction of the pressure difference, and would not be able to vibrate properly. The design device that enables this pressure equalization to be achieved is the Eustachian tube; its presence means that air on each side of the eardrum is in communication and will, therefore, be at the same pressure. The crucial importance of this tube is revealed when it becomes blocked — when we have a cold or when rapid air pressure changes are experienced, as in an airplane. The resulting unequalized pressures in the ear cause pain and a temporary mild hearing loss.

The other subtle function of the components of the middle ear is partly a protective one. Transmission of energy through the middle ear can be modified by middle ear muscles. The tensor tympani muscle pulls at the base of the long arm of the malleus and increases tension in the eardrum. The stapedius muscle pulls on the neck of the stapes at right angles to the "piston" axis of the bone. When this muscle does contract, it tends to immobilize the footplate region of the stapes.

A Protective Reflex

Both these muscular actions increase the stiffness of the ossicle chain and greatly reduce the efficiency of energy transfer through the middle ear, particularly of sounds at frequencies below 2000 Hz. The attenuation may be down to one thousandth of the

25

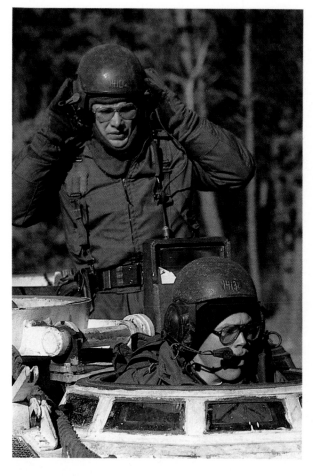

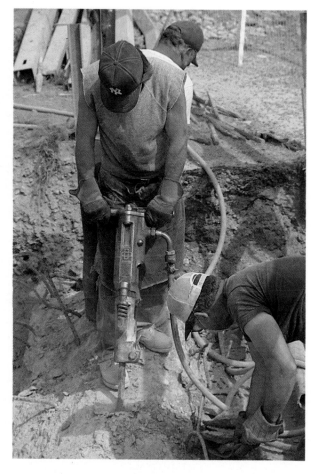

previous level for some frequencies. Why should this beautifully designed amplifier system suddenly want to "turn down" its amplification by the use of these muscles? One reason is probably to protect the inner ear from sudden, very loud sounds, which can irreparably damage the receptor cells within the cochlea. In the normal ear, the tensor tympani and the stapedius muscles contract automatically in response to sounds over 80 decibels received by either ear. This response begins within 15 to 150 milliseconds of reception of the loud noise starting, and maximum protection is produced within some 100 to 500 milliseconds. By reacting so quickly, the muscle reflexes protect the receptor cells against intense sounds in the frequency range below 2000 Hz. Unfortunately, the reflex is not quick enough to protect the ears against the damaging effects of, for example, the sound of

close gunfire. Such explosive sound increases peak too quickly for the muscles to react in time.

Having journeyed far into the inner spaces of the human auditory system through the outer and middle ears, we have now reached the threshold of the inner ear — the oval window. On the far side of that window is the inner ear, a tiny concentration of receptor structures of amazing complexity. The meandering convolutions of its many parts may seem designed to tax the agility of the human brain as much as anything.

The vestibular apparatus, which occupies much of the inner ear's bulk, has nothing to do with sound perception. The hair cells (receptor cells) of the vestibular labyrinth provide the brain with information on the position of the head relative to gravity. They also signal angular and linear movements of the head; that is, turning movements and

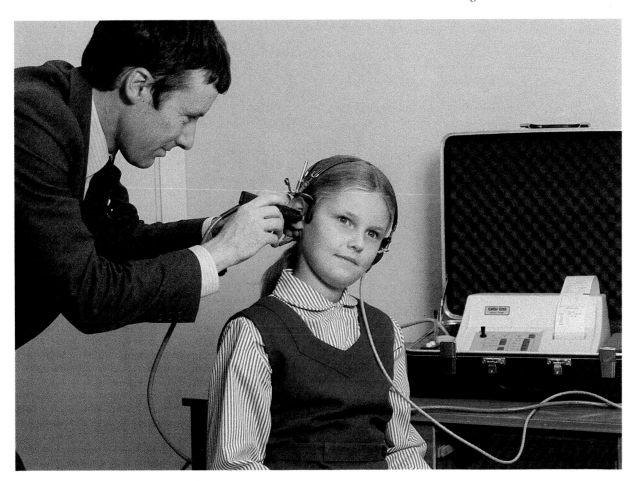

movements in a single direction. Hair cells in the three semicircular canals of each ear are the main receptors for turning (angular) acceleration. At a nonconscious, reflex level, their stimulation brings about appropriate muscle activities in the eyes, neck, limbs and vertebral column to make compensations for such turning.

So-called otolith receptor cells in other parts of the vestibular labyrinth detect the direction of gravity and straight-line movements; again, these have reflex connections with appropriate compensatory muscle systems. The nervous signals pass from the vestibular apparatus to the brain along the vestibular branch of the VIIIth cranial nerve. Overall, the functions of these nerve impulses are twofold. First, they relate to the control of balance, a crucial task for an animal walking on only two limbs as man does. Second, they are essential in the co-

ordination of the eye and head movement, so visual capacity is optimized while the head is moving.

The other half of the labyrinth, the portion dominated by the cochlea, is the true seat of human hearing abilities and, as such, our main concern here. Both the vestibular and cochlear sections are contained in a single closed system of interconnecting ducts and chambers called the membranous labyrinth. The development of this structure during the embryonic and fetal periods of a baby in the womb is a fascinating story. Only some eighteen days into development, even before the brain has rolled itself into a closed organ system, a group of surface, epithelial cells on each side of the head of the embryo starts to dimple. Each one of these cell groups, called the otic placodes, forms a hollow sphere of cells, the otic vesicle, as it moves into the substance of the head. This simple bubble of cells is

The extraordinary complex route by which vibrations pass from the stapes bone to the organ of Corti are shown in this stylized image of the cochlear region of the inner ear. Vibrations of the footplate of the stapes transmit vibrations to the fluid contents of the scala vestibuli. These perturbations pass up the "snail-shell" shape of the cochlea, change their direction at the apex of the cochlea (the helicotrema) and descend the spiral by way of the scala tympani. Hair cell receptors in the organ of Corti are stimulated by the vibrations in these fluid-filled passageways to produce nerve impulses, which pass to the brain via the cochlear nerve.

THE COCHLEA

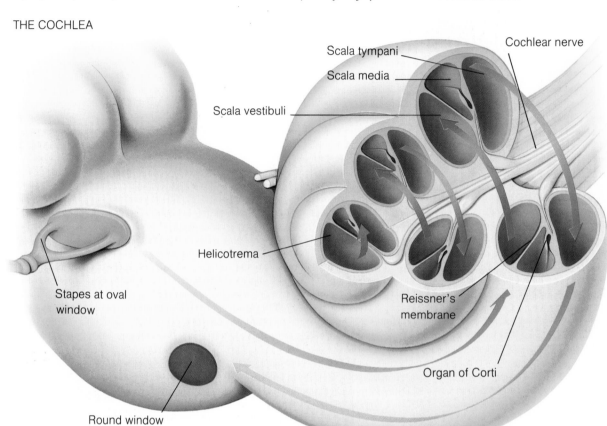

Scala tympani

Scala media

Cochlear nerve

Scala vestibuli

Helicotrema

Reissner's membrane

Organ of Corti

Stapes at oval window

Round window

destined, after contortions that would make a glass-blower gasp with admiration, to make all the multifarious parts of the membranous labyrinth.

At various locations over the inner surface of the final labyrinth system, receptor hair cells point inward and produce nerve impulses in the nerve fibers associated with them, when the hairs at their tips are moved or bent. Such stimulation is typically caused when the fluid contents of the labyrinth — the endolymph — moves relative to the hairs. Stimulation of the hairs in the vestibular apparatus signals gravitational orientation of movements; stimulation of the hair cells in the cochlea signals the presence of sounds.

Like the rest of the membranous labyrinth, the cochlear part is enclosed, like a coiled snake in a coiled tunnel, in a bony cavity — the bony labyrinth. The "coiled snake," which contains fluid (endolymph) and the hair cells of the cochlea, is known as the scala media or the cochlear duct. The cell systems within it, which enable auditory nerve impulses to be produced, are together called the organ of Corti, after their discoverer. The oval window, with its connections to the footplate of the stapes, is a membrane that separates the air of the middle ear from the liquid in the "snake's tunnel," a fluid different from endolymph called perilymph. Movements of the oval window, caused by sounds activating the ossicle chain, set up fluid pressure changes in the perilymph.

The track of these pressure changes is bizarre because of the detailed internal anatomy of the bony and membranous tubes. At any point in the two and a half turns of the snail-shaped cochlea, the "snake" (that is, the membranous tube or cochlear duct) is sandwiched between two different perilymph-filled spaces. Above is the scala vestibuli, below the scala tympani. It is the perilymph

28

Alfonso Corti

Investigator of the Inner Ear

Alfonso Giacomo Gaspare Corti was born in 1822 at Gambarana, near Pavia, Italy, the heir to a noble family of Lombardy, which had, however, seen better days. Corti appears to have fallen under the spell of his father's scientific interests and, at the age of nineteen, went to medical school in Pavia. But he did not finish his course because, four years later, he decided to enrol as a student at Vienna University, where the most famous professors were teaching. Graduating in 1847, he remained at Vienna as assistant to Professor Joseph Hyrel at the Institute of Anatomy.

The sensory organs quickly became Corti's favorite subject, so when Hyrel recommended Corti should investigate the structure of the inner ear, he began at once. Unfortunately, his researches were cut short by war between Austria and the Kingdom of Sardinia — as the Piedmontese realm of his home was then called. So Corti moved to Switzerland, where in Zürich, in 1849, he began his own microscopic studies.

In January 1850, Corti went to Würzburg, Germany, where he learned normal histology in only two months from the master anatomist Albert Kölliker. It was here that Corti

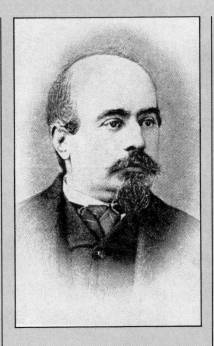

investigated the retina of the eye and discovered how its nerve cells connect with the fibers of the optic nerve.

All the while, Corti had been continuing with his study of the inner ear, which proved fruitless until he visited the Harting Observatorium in Utrecht, Holland, where Harting showed him how to prepare moist specimens of the membranous labyrinth of the cochlea properly. Within a year, Corti had completed the brilliant work which revealed the acoustic receptor of the inner ear. For the first time, scientists could look at drawings and microscope

slides of the organ of hearing, later, in his honor, called 'the organ of Corti' by Kölliker.

This work Corti performed partly in Würzburg and partly in Paris. He studied the cochleas of various animals always using the freshest possible material. His observations were all the more remarkable because he could use only pieces of membranous cochlea — sometimes a few millimeters thick — instead of fine sections. He also discovered the method of staining slides with carmine solution — a red cochineal dye that enabled him to distinguish the individual components of the organ: the sensory cells, the tectorial membrane, the spiral ganglion and the pillars of corti.

He published his results in Paris in 1851, the same year that Ernst Reissner (1824–1878) described the vestibular membrane of the cochlea. Only six years later, Hermann von Helmholtz published the first draft of his resonance theory of hearing, which was based upon the discoveries of Corti.

Pressing family matters forced Corti to return to Turin almost at once and, while he occasionally published some inconclusive work, he disappeared from the scientific scene and died in 1876.

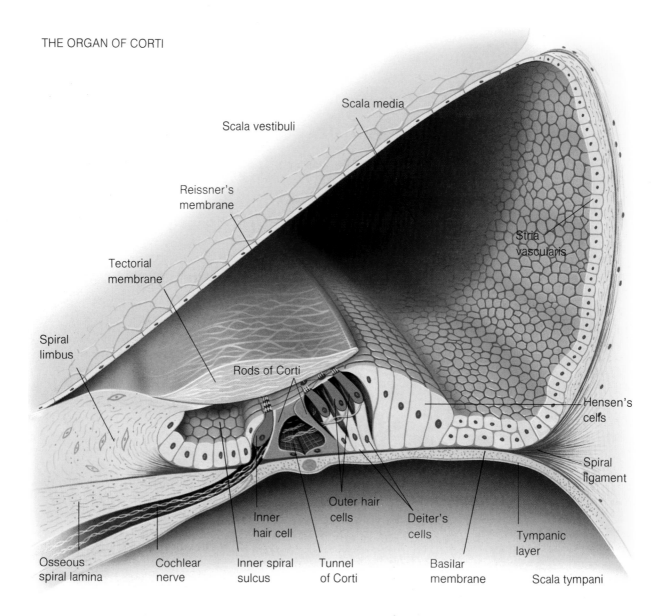

Scala media

Scala vestibuli

Reissner's membrane

Tectorial membrane

Stria vascularis

Spiral limbus

Rods of Corti

Hensen's cells

Spiral ligament

Inner hair cell

Outer hair cells

Deiter's cells

Tympanic layer

Osseous spiral lamina

Cochlear nerve

Inner spiral sulcus

Tunnel of Corti

Basilar membrane

Scala tympani

in the former which is perturbed by the movements of the oval window, set in the wall of the bony labyrinth near the base of the "snail shell" of the cochlea. The pressure changes pass from base to apex of the "snail" in the scala vestibuli and then down the "helter-skelter," again from apex to base, via the scala tympani. The two scalae interconnect at the apex of the helical shell-shape. A quite separate membranous partition, the round window, separates the lower end of the scala tympani space from the middle ear.

It has been a long descriptive track from the eardrum to the cochlea, but the energy transfer processes of the acoustic part of the ear are now approaching their natural conclusion. To summarize the phases of the transfer so far: first, sound-produced air pressure changes in the ear canal set up mechanical vibrations of the eardrum. These, with considerable mechanical amplification, pass along the ossicle chain to the oval window. The movements of the window set up corresponding vibrations in the perilymph fluid of the bony chamber of the cochlea. Sandwiched between two interconnected tubes of the vibrating perilymph lies the cochlear duct which houses the organ of Corti and the acoustic hair cells. With the coupling of perilymph pressure changes to bending or shearing movements of the receptor cell hairs, the original sound stimulus is brought to the outposts of the nervous system, but how is this coupling achieved?

Fluctuations in pressure in the perilymph of the scala vestibuli efficiently induce corresponding pressure changes in the endolymph fluid of the cochlear duct because the two fluid-filled spaces are separated by only a thin membrane (Reissner's membrane). Endolymph pressure changes cause vibrations in the lower bounding membrane of the cochlear duct, the all-important basilar membrane. Attached to its upper surface are the acoustic hair cells — 12,000 or so outer hair cells and 3,500 inner hair cells in the human cochlea.

The outer hair cells have their receptor hairs embedded in a flap, the tectorial membrane, which sticks out into the endolymph-filled cochlear duct. The inner hair cells do not have their tips restricted in this way. Both types of receptor cell, however, can be stimulated when the basilar membrane moves up and down under the influence of perilymphatic pressure changes.

The system of coupling between the incoming sound stimuli and the receptor cells so far described explains only how we register the presence of sound. It does nothing to explain loudness and pitch sensitivity. The answer to this and related questions lies in the precise types of vibration set up in the basilar membrane by sounds and in the behavior of individual receptor cells.

Patterns of Membrane Movement

Much of the knowledge of these crucial areas of hearing physiology stems from the pioneering work of the Hungarian scientist Georg von Békésy. A prolific and innovative worker, he demonstrated how sound waves of different intensity and frequency had specifically different effects on the vibration patterns of the basilar membrane. The changing stiffness and width of the membrane, from base to apex of the cochlear helix, play an important part in inducing these patterns. The waves in the basilar membrane are so-called traveling waves, which propagate from the base to apex of the cochlea. Since the basilar membrane becomes floppier and wider progressively from base to apex, high-frequency sounds tend to vibrate the basilar membrane maximally at its base, low-frequency sounds to produce the largest membrane movements at the apex.

This graded response of the membrane to sounds of different frequency shows the way in which the ear extracts information about pitch from the incoming sound signals. It appears that the basilar membrane, by having its different zones sharply

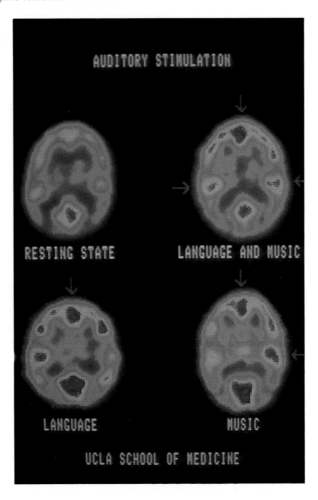

Experimental brain scans by a process known as PCT, or Positron Computed Tomography, reveal which parts of the brain are activated when a person perceives sound. The subject is injected with a radioactive substance similar to glucose, the brain's chief source of fuel. While the patient is exposed to various types of sound, the machine scans sections of the brain and shows up areas of glucose consumption, corresponding to brain activity, as dark regions. The process reveals interesting differences in the areas affected by the stimuli.

Holding a conch shell to her ear, this little girl marvels as she seems to hear the pounding sea within it. In fact, the shell is acting like a tiny echo chamber. Its wide mouth collects the low level sounds in the vicinity and intensifies them within its narrow passages. Because the inner surfaces of the shell are hard and shiny, little of the sound is absorbed, and it remains trapped inside the shell, creating echoes as it bounces from surface to surface until all its energy is dissipated. These booming echoes, so reminiscent of the sea, are the source of the conch shell's seemingly magic song.

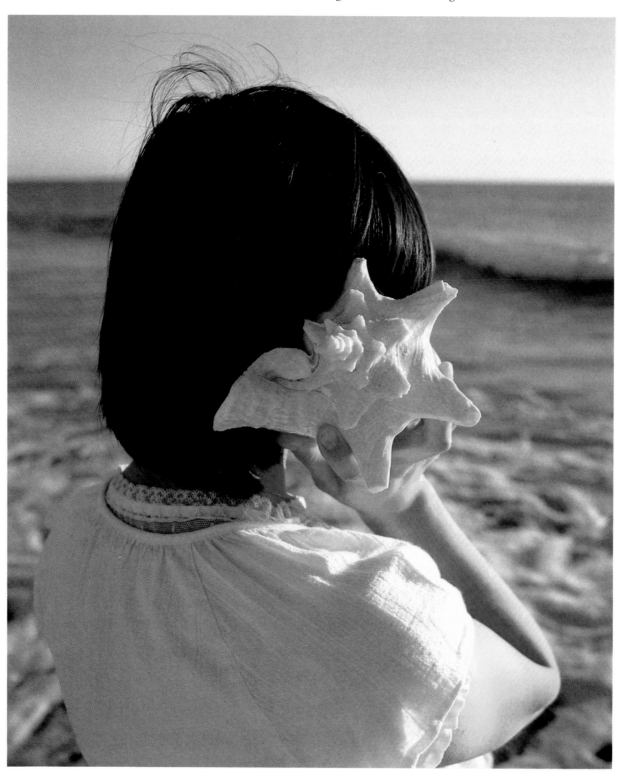

"tuned" to respond maximally to different sound frequencies, is able selectively to stimulate only a small subpopulation of hair cells when a particular note is received. Similarly, as the extent of membrane movement is also related to the intensity of the sound input, membrane movements, when translated into receptor cell activity, will be able to signal information about loudness as well.

The studies of von Békésy and others have shown that the peak movements of the basilar membrane are some thirty times greater in size than those of the stapes footplate. They are, even so, exceedingly small, measuring only some 10 to 100 nanometers at high sound intensities — one nanometer is a millionth of a millimeter.

Pathway to the Brain

The exact mechanism by which the basilar membrane movements excite the hair cells is the subject of lively controversy and many theories. It is likely, though, that bending or shearing movements of the hairs relative to the apex of the cell induces a change in the difference in electrical charge between the contents of the cell and its surroundings. This change, technically a depolarization, will in turn stimulate the release of a chemical transmitter substance, probably glutamic acid, at the base of the cell. The substance initiates a nerve impulse in the sensory nerve that has connections with the hair cells. Recordings from individual nerve axons in the auditory portion of cranial nerve VIII show that individual fibers demonstrate great selectivity in their firing patterns, in response to stimuli of different intensity and frequency. For low-intensity stimuli, each fiber has only a single frequency to which it will respond with nerve impulses. As the intensity of the stimulus is increased, a wider and wider band of frequencies around the initial preferred one will be able to induce some sort of response in the nerve axon.

The mechanisms that form the working basis of our auditory system, described above, ensure that stimulus frequency becomes encoded according to the position on the basilar membrane at which hair cells are stimulated. This pattern of information coding is preserved at the level of the many small nerve "nuclei," which collect together sensory fibers from small sectors of the cochlea. The same

Dumb Speech *or* Language *of the* Fingers.

Note for (h) and (r) let the Finger be brought from one end of the Line where it is set, to the other end thereof.

Publish'd according to Act of Parliament, for J. Hinton at the King's Arms, in S.t Paul's Church Yard, London. 1748.

quasi-spatial patterning standing for frequency is maintained at the progressively higher levels of the nervous system that process auditory data. This arrangement is certainly present in the brain stem, midbrain, thalamic and auditory cortex levels.

At the auditory cortex, our journey through the sensory system from sound stimulus to perception is complete. Once in the realm of the conscious mind, the sound can be referred to in terms of pitch and loudness: the mind's interpretation of frequency and intensity respectively. Before moving on to look at the ways in which these sophisticated hearing abilities fit into the context of human existence, clap your hands once. The sound is instantly heard, yet think of the processes it has gone through in order to be heard: processes that take pages to describe, a fraction of a second to operate.

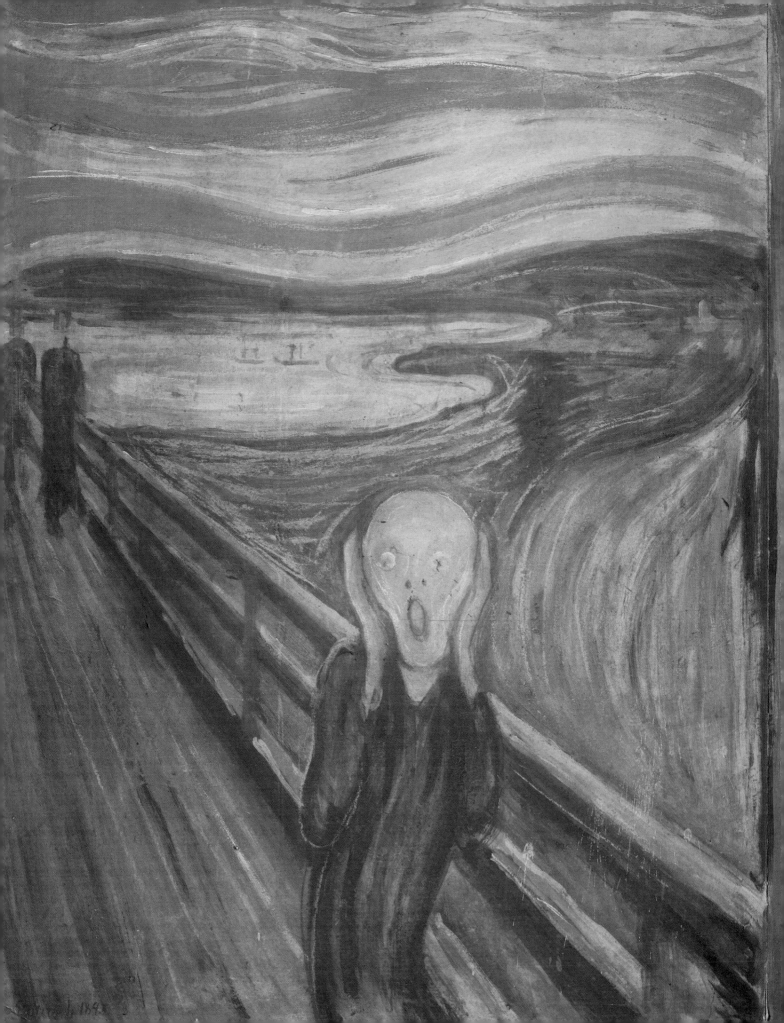

Chapter 2

Sound and Hearing

So far we have spent a considerable amount of time describing the nature of sound stimuli and the structure and mechanics of the ear to intercept those stimuli. But physiological responses of the auditory system tell us little about what is actually perceived. Wavelengths do not have any intrinsic sound until we catch them with our ears and process them with our brains. What we perceive with our ears, as with our eyes or our noses, is dependent upon how we handle the incoming information. The field of psychophysics deals with the procedures and techniques used to obtain answers from people to questions such as, "What do you respond to?" It thus embraces the relationship between physical and psychological aspects of a stimulus and has two main approaches.

The first is to present a subject with two different stimuli and ask him if he can discriminate between them; the second involves the experimenter asking the subject about the stimuli — is one louder, stronger, more or less pleasant, than another? From his observations on a great many subjects, the experimenter can build a picture of the "normal" human response to the stimulus and then use this as the baseline to determine perceptual malfunction of the sensory system. The field of auditory psychophysics is quite well developed, much more so than that of gustatory or olfactory psychophysics, although the same approaches apply.

Thresholds of Human Audibility

The first matter that must be considered is that of audibility: everybody has their own threshold of audibility for each frequency of sound. A graph displaying the lowest sound intensity required to detect a sound of various frequencies is called an audiogram. To obtain an audiogram, the subject wears earphones, through which pure tones of known intensity may be delivered. The sound pressure level, at which the sound is barely audible, is measured in decibels. The American National

The minimum level at which a sound can be heard depends on its frequency and is less in the middle of our hearing range than at either end. For example, a tone of 5000 Hz must be of 10 decibels to be heard (below).

Conversational speech spans the frequency range 50 to 8000 Hz. Compare this to the range of a piano — where C4 is middle C — of 30 to 4000 Hz. Consonants use more of the range than vowels and occupy

the higher levels, but there is no difference in the frequencies produced by men and women. Laryngeal sounds (vowels), however, occupy the lower part of the range and differ in male and female voices (right).

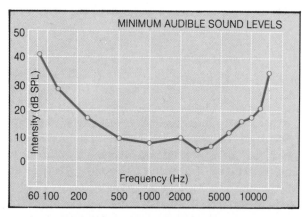

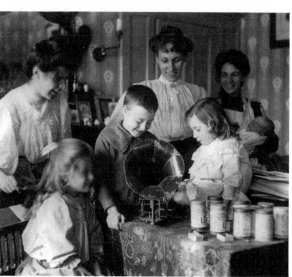

In 1877, Thomas Edison discovered that the pressure patterns of sound waves could be translated by a metal stylus into permanent patterns on tinfoil and then replayed by passing the stylus back over the grooves. He had invented the phonograph. Immediately adopted by an enthusiastic public, the machine was a huge success and, by the early twentieth century, improved models were selling in their thousands for the playing of recorded material in the home. Seen by some as a mixed blessing, the age of recorded sound had arrived.

Standards Institute (ANSI) published normative data in 1969 that is still in use today.

Human beings are maximally sensitive to frequencies of 1000 to 3000 Hz, though we can detect tones over the range of approximately 20 Hz to 20,000 Hz. At frequencies above and below our most sensitive range, we have higher thresholds, that is, the sounds need to be louder for us to hear them. Extremely low sounds, such as that emerging from a 32-foot organ pipe, and extremely high sounds, such as high-pitched bells and the top notes on a piano, may require intensities four or five times greater than those required for the perception of tones at the frequency of the human voice. A sound with a frequency of about 1000 Hz (for example, the C two octaves above Middle C on the piano) at 150 decibels (dB SPL) is so intense that the subject feels real pain. So we can summarize the capability of human hearing by saying that we are sensitive to a frequency range of about 20,000 Hz and an intensity range of some 150 decibels.

Filtering Sound

In a very real sense, the sort of tests used to determine audibility are quite artificial, since we seldom if ever encounter simple, pure tones. Because they consist of a mixture of tones of differing frequencies, most sounds we hear are termed complex sounds. If the components of a complex sound are sufficiently far apart in frequency, we can hear them as separate notes, such as the notes in a chord. But if they are close together, we hear them as one note. Speech is an excellent example of a stream of complex sounds, and if we are to resolve — and, therefore, understand — speech we must analyze sounds that are present simultaneously. The ear acts as a bank of hypothetical filters, and psychophysical estimates of the "shape" of these filters resembles those of the frequency threshold curves of the cochlear nerve fiber.

This has been discovered by conducting experiments in which a wide bandwidth of sound is presented alongside a signal tone; this tone is thus shrouded in unimportant sounds, or noise. The threshold for detection of this tone can be determined in the presence of this noise. As the bandwidth of noise is narrowed, a critical point is reached, when the intensity level suddenly falls, at

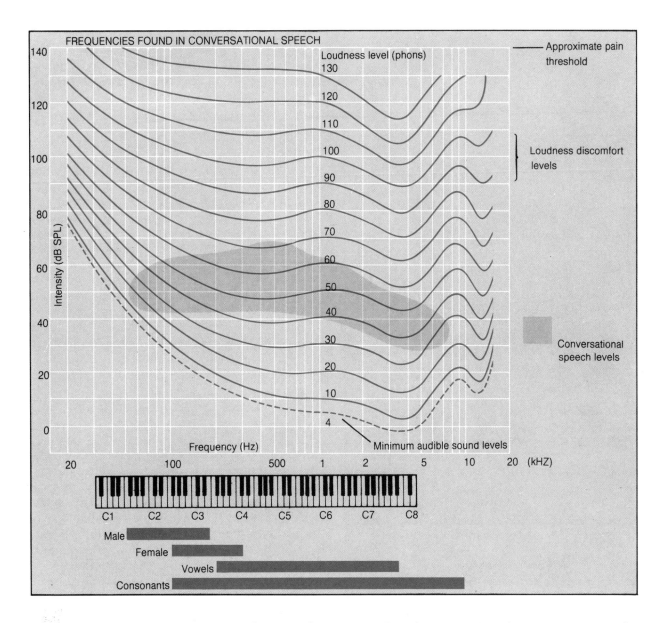

FREQUENCIES FOUND IN CONVERSATIONAL SPEECH

Approximate pain threshold

Loudness level (phons)
130
120
110
100
90
80
70
60
50
40
30
20
10
4

Loudness discomfort levels

Conversational speech levels

Minimum audible sound levels

Intensity (dB SPL)

140
120
100
80
60
40
20
0

Frequency (Hz)

20   100   500   1   2   5   10   20   (kHZ)

C1   C2   C3   C4   C5   C6   C7   C8

Male
Female
Vowels
Consonants

which the signal tone can be detected among the noise. In other words, the signal suddenly becomes easier to detect among the noise. So when you are talking to somebody, among the clatter of office or subway noise, your brain is rapidly deploying filter after filter — depending on the change of frequency of the speaker's voice — so the signal-to-noise ratio is at its highest.

Audiologists think that the filtering process starts in the cochlear nerve, whose fibers appear to act, as a first approximation, as linear filters. So long as a complex sound like speech contains frequency components separated by frequencies greater than the amount of filtering provided by these fibers, then, in theory, each component can be resolved. At fairly low frequencies, between 60 and 1000 Hz, we can discriminate frequencies as little as 2 Hz

apart. But above 1000 Hz, the separation must be much greater. This is further complicated by the fact that quieter sounds are more difficult to discriminate than louder ones and require separation of more than 2 Hz. At 4000 Hz, for instance, a 10 decibel sound requires to be separated by 24 Hz from another for discrimination. At 60 decibels, however, 16 Hz is all that is required for us to be able to tell two tones apart.

The Resonance Theory of Pitch

All this brings us to a consideration of pitch, and what a complex subject it is! When we relax in the concert hall and let the orchestral cadences flow over us, our ability to discriminate pitch is working overtime. We can tell in a flash if one instrument among a hundred or so on the platform is not

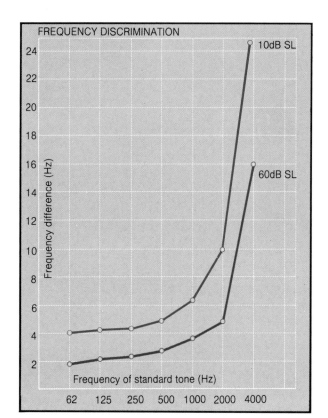

FREQUENCY DISCRIMINATION

10dB SL

60dB SL

Frequency difference (Hz)

Frequency of standard tone (Hz)

62 125 250 500 1000 2000 4000

If two tones with frequencies close together are heard simultaneously, the louder the tones are, the easier it is to discriminate between them. As the frequencies of the tones rise, the human ear becomes less able to differentiate one tone from another. The graph shows curves for two loudnesses of noise — 10 decibels and 60 decibels. Over the range 62 to 1000 Hz, a difference in frequency of at least 4 to 6 Hz is required for the discrimination of the tones when the sound level is 10 decibels, but only half this is needed when the sound is louder. At 2000 Hz, the frequency difference must be 14 Hz at 10 decibels and 6 Hz at 60 decibels. At higher pitches, the frequency difference needs to be still greater.

holding the pitch it should. Trained musicians know that the pitch of a tone is not simply a function of frequency, though this is the most important component of pitch; sound intensity, too, affects pitch in a complex manner that is not well understood.

Two kinds of theory have been put forward to explain the phenomenon of pitch. The first is called the "place" or "resonance" theory and it was propounded by Hermann von Helmholtz in 1857. He observed that the basilar membrane of the organ of Corti was composed of fibers running radially, and that the width of the membrane increased from the base of the cochlear spiral to its apex. Helmholtz thought the membrane was under tension and that the taut fibers could act as stretched strings. He assumed that each would respond to an individual frequency, just as a resonator will resonate if it stands in the path of its particular frequency.

The Vibrating Membrane

How this works can be demonstrated by taking a vibrating tuning fork, which is producing a constant pure tone of a single frequency, and moving it slowly over the stretched strings of a piano. If the fork is producing C, the C strings will vibrate, and the piano will sing in sympathy. Everything is able to resonate and everything has its own resonating frequency. In fact, this is the principle upon which a microwave oven works: when you put a potato into the oven and switch on, waves of very short wavelength bombard the potato and cause the water molecules to vibrate. These are very much smaller than the carbohydrate molecules that comprise the rest of the potato, so the flesh of the potato does not resonate. If it did, there would be little potato left, for it would be blasted into millions of fragments. The result is that the excitement caused in the water molecules generates a lot of heat and so the potato is cooked. (Recall that when a sound wave travels through the air, molecules are excited and the air heats up very slightly.)

To return to the pitch theory: Helmholtz argued that the shorter fibers under most tension at the base of the cochlea would respond to high frequencies, giving the perception of high pitch, while the slacker fibers at its apex would vibrate in sympathy, with lower frequencies, and transmit the impression of bass notes. Helmholtz refined his

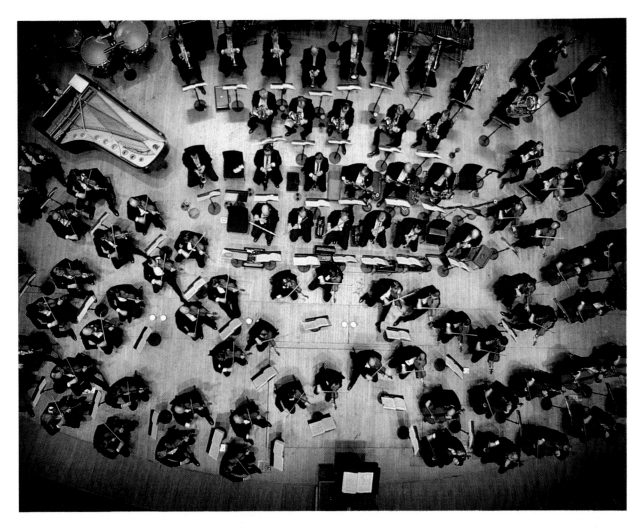

theory by stating that the strength of the stimulus would be represented by the magnitude of the membrane vibration, and this would then determine the magnitude of the nerve response. Thus the essence of Helmholtz's theory was that the sensation of pitch depended upon the place along the basilar membrane that responded to the stimulus.

For a number of years Helmholtz's theory attracted a lot of interest, but gradually its shortcomings emerged. First, it was found that the basilar membrane is not under significant tension, so the fibers are not stretched and thus could not. resonate. Second, calculations made on actual fibers revealed that their length and mass are such that, if they did resonate, they would respond to only a small range of the total 20,000 Hz or so that we can hear.

Third, and by analogy with string instruments such as the piano, it was argued that if a resonator is used for discrimination of a very narrow range of frequencies and over a very short period, it must be highly damped, so as to stop its vibrations once the

sound has been perceived. Psychophysical experiments reveal that the frequency discrimination of the ear is simply too good for the operation of a strong damper, and, in any case, there is no anatomical evidence of muscles or other structures which could damp a vibrating membrane. Finally, it was pointed out in the first part of the twentieth century by the British Lord Adrian, winner of the Nobel Prize for Physiology and Medicine, that nerves respond according to an all-or-nothing principle and that their response is not graded with intensity of stimulus.

Lord Rutherford and "Nerve Vibrations"

Toward the end of the nineteenth century, the British physicist Lord Rutherford ignored the resonance theory and, in its place, proposed that the entire organ of Corti was activated by all perceived frequencies and that the particular characteristics of the sound were directly represented in what he termed "nerve vibrations." He proposed that a single nerve could simultaneously represent

Georg von Békésy

Discoverer of the "Traveling Wave"

No scientist has contributed more to the understanding of how our ears work than Georg von Békésy. His precise and ingenious mind solved many of the riddles of hearing.

Born in 1899, in Budapest, Hungary, he first became fascinated by the power of sound when he heard, as a boy, the high-pitched notes of gypsy music. The son of a diplomat, he went to school in a number of European cities, studied chemistry at the University of Berne, Switzerland and finally received his Ph.D in physics from the University of Budapest, in 1923.

The Hungarian Telephone Research Laboratory immediately gave him the task of improving the telephone system, especially the long-distance network. He started to study the human ear to determine whether the quality of its hearing warranted significant improvements in the telephone, and was prompted by the excellence of the ear's ability to hear to discover how it really worked.

Scientists had known for some time that vibrations of the basilar membrane in the cochlea are responsible for transmitting information about sound to the brain. Von Békésy realized that each of these

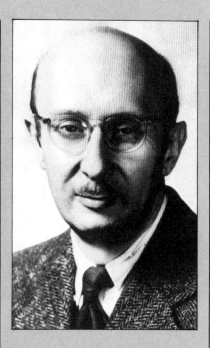

theories made basic assumptions about the physical properties of the membrane — its elasticity, shape and friction, for example — so he examined the basilar membranes from various animals and constructed models to imitate them.

In 1928, he proposed that sound waves, transmitted via the eardrum and the bones of the middle ear to the oval window, set up traveling waves in the basilar membrane. Within twenty years he had proved it beyond doubt.

In 1946, von Békésy left Hungary, spent a year working in Stockholm and, in 1949,

became a senior research fellow at the Psycho-Acoustic Laboratory at Harvard. Here he built a model which, it was reported in 1958, allowed the skin to "hear." The model consisted of a water-filled plastic bag with a membrane twelve inches long, which, when stimulated, exhibited the same traveling waves as those in the cochlea. By placing his forearm against this model, von Békésy sensed the vibrations as they traveled along the membrane. Surprisingly, he sensed the peak of the vibration in a section of the membrane only three-quarters to one inch long; when the frequency of stimulation was increased, the section of sensed vibration moved toward the end representing the oval window of the cochlea. When the frequency was decreased, the section moved the other way.

Von Békésy had discovered, at last, that different frequencies of sound are analyzed by the cochlea at different locations along the basilar membrane. For this and other discoveries concerning the physical mechanisms of stimulation within the cochlea, in 1961, von Békésy became the first physicist to win the Nobel Prize for Physiology and Medicine.

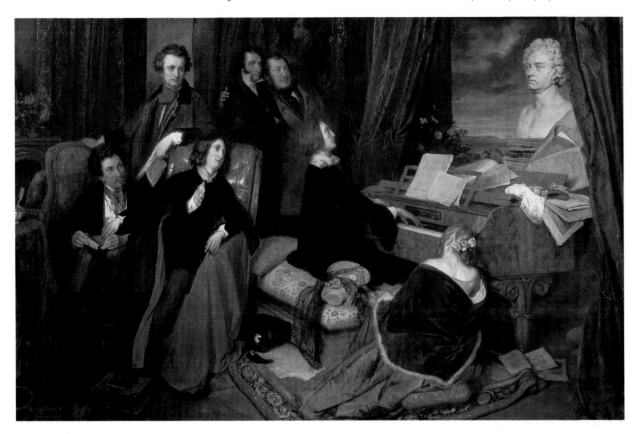

the parameters of the sound by slight variations in the magnitude, shape and frequency of its evoked action potential. The brain would then unscramble this complex impulse, leaving the subject with a clear indication of pitch, intensity and general sound quality.

Once again, the basic information on how nerves work, put forth by Lord Adrian, makes the theory untenable, since the magnitude and shape of the nerve fiber's action potential is constant. Additionally, nerve physiologists soon showed that nerve impulses could be produced at rates of up to a maximum of 500 per second: if frequency of pitch were to be coded by the rate of impulse production, then a tone of 500 Hz (or 500 cycles per second) would be the highest perceptible. But since we know that humans perceive sounds up to 20,000 Hz, this theory does not seem capable of fully explaining pitch perception.

In 1928, the Hungarian Georg von Békésy put forward his case for the traveling wave theory, to explain mechanically how the cochlea could work. His careful measurements revealed that sounds below 20 Hz produced no vibrations in the basilar membrane. Between this and 2000 Hz, the entire membrane vibrated, and above 2000 Hz only a restricted part of the membrane did so. Notice that von Békésy stated that the vibration was of only "part" of the membrane — not just of a single fiber.

The "Volley" Theory

Von Békésy's ideas were extended in 1949, when the American otologist E. G. Wever combined Rutherford's and von Békésy's theories. Wever's studies led him to suggest that at between 20 Hz and 400 Hz individual nerve fibers in the cochlear nerve can respond to each 1 Hz of tone, so they will fire off their impulse once in each cycle, or Hertz of tone. The intensity of the tone would, therefore, be represented by the *number* of neurons firing once for every Hertz of tone.

For frequencies above 400 Hz and up to 5000 Hz,

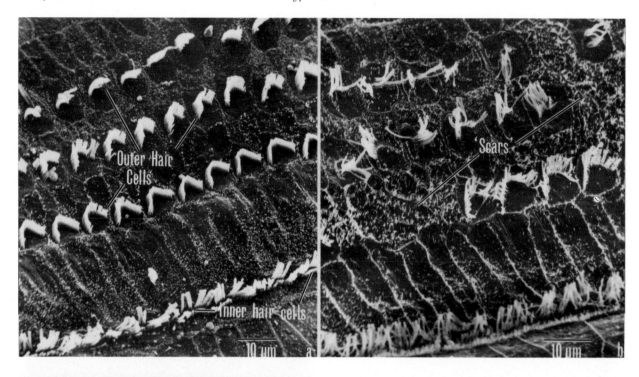

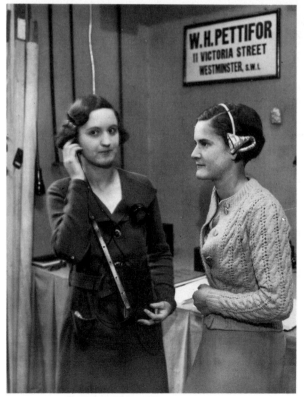

a more complex situation exists. Although the rate at which nerve fibers can fire their impulses is limited to 500 per second, Wever suggested that they stagger their response and may respond to every third, fourth or fifth cycle of the tone. This theory is called the ''volley'' theory because the response of the *whole nerve* involves having its neurons fire in volleys in order to increase the frequency of response and thereby represent higher frequencies. Intensity continues to be represented by the number of fibers contributing to each synchronous burst within the cochlear nerve; but as the intensity increases, the fibers are said to fire earlier in their ''resting period'' between firings. Thus, instead of firing, they contribute to increase the number of impulses each second in each volley in the whole nerve. (The human audiogram shows that intensity needs to be increased for high-pitch perception.) For frequencies above 5000 Hz, Wever argued that the place principle operated, with sound intensity coded in number of impulses per second.

Pitch perception is not yet fully understood. On present evidence, it seems likely that a volley-type mechanism operates for low-frequency sounds (approximately 20 Hz to 1000 Hz or so) and that a

A complex stimulus of tones of 700, 800, 900 and 1000 Hz, delivered at 10 millisecond intervals, is heard as a tone of only 100 Hz because this is the frequency associated with a 10 millisecond period. Similarly, pulsed tones produce perceived frequencies according to their periodicity. Thus, for a pulse with a period of 0.5 milliseconds the loudest perceived tone is at 2000 Hz with subsidiary components at 6000, 10,000 and 14,000 Hz.

traveling wave comes into operation from about 1000 Hz up to about 5000 Hz (but with some interaction of the volley theory), while above 5000 Hz, the traveling wave alone is responsible for pitch perception. We should note that these theories may yet be stood on their heads, for there is much active research going on in this area, and more refined observations are being made all the time.

The Missing Fundamental

Theory is all very well, but of course, in practice, things must be more complex. Seldom do we hear pure tones of single frequencies. Usually we hear complex sounds containing several components, and, in particular, we hear sounds which carry subsidiary tones at double and triple frequencies to the tone we think we are perceiving. These are called the harmonics: in this instance, the second and third harmonics of the fundamental, or first harmonic. The listener is unaware that he is hearing a number of different frequencies, for he thinks he is hearing just the fundamental.

It has been shown by experimentation that some harmonics can be filtered out without altering the perceived pitch of a note. Amazingly, even the fundamental can be filtered out, and the listener reports he still hears it. This has been graphically termed "the case of the missing fundamental," and it is much more common than one might imagine. The oboe, for instance, that wonderful reedy upholder of the plaintive line in music, is an instrument in which little sound energy is produced at the frequency corresponding to the pitch heard.

The phenomenon is also observed with church bells. When a bell is struck by the clapper, a series of frequencies is produced above and below the fundamental. In the case of one particular bell, the following frequencies were recorded by instrumentation: 293.7 Hz; 440.0 Hz; 587.3 Hz; 784.0 Hz; and 987.8 Hz. The pitch perceived by the listener was none of these, but 493.9 Hz — exactly an octave below the highest component actually produced by the vibrating bell. Studies such as these indicate that pitch perception is more complex than the theory suggests and that there exist mechanisms yet undiscovered.

The time structure of the waveform may also play a part in pitch perception. It has been demonstrated

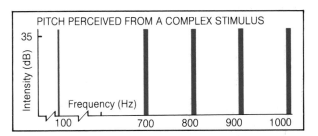

PITCH PERCEIVED FROM A COMPLEX STIMULUS

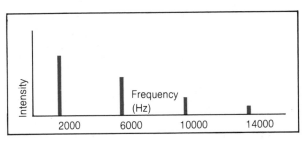

PITCHES PERCEIVED FROM A 0.5 MILLISECOND PULSE

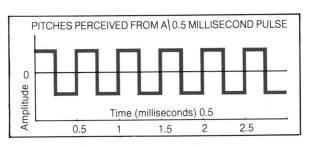

that people hear a 100 Hz pitch when presented with a complex sound consisting of just 700, 800, 900 and 1000 Hz. Since the sound contains no energy at 100 Hz, why is a pitch of 100 Hz heard? These four tones are all harmonics of 100 Hz, and, in fact, 100 Hz is the highest frequency for which these tones are harmonically related. When the waveform of this complex sound is examined, it turns out that the time interval between major peaks of energy is 10 milliseconds. A period of 10 milliseconds corresponds to a frequency of 100 Hz, so it appears that listeners hear this missing fundamental because of the 10 millisecond periodicity in the waveform. It has been shown that any sound stimulus with a periodic waveform has a perceived pitch equal to the reciprocal of its periodicity. Thus if a complex sound has a 2 millisecond periodicity, the perceived pitch will be 500 Hz, and, if it has a 0.5 millisecond periodicity, it will have a 2000 Hz pitch.

Sometimes we hear tones which we know are distorted, and the reason for the distortion is

As a fast car passes a stationary observer, the perceived pitch of its engine seems to decrease, yet to the driver it remains constant. This change of pitch is called the Doppler effect and is caused by the sound waves that come from the car bunching up as it approaches, so pushing up the pitch, and stretching out as it recedes, thus lowering the pitch. The faster the car the greater the change in pitch.

THE DOPPLER EFFECT

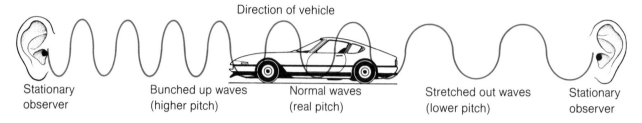

Direction of vehicle

Stationary observer

Bunched up waves (higher pitch)

Normal waves (real pitch)

Stretched out waves (lower pitch)

Stationary observer

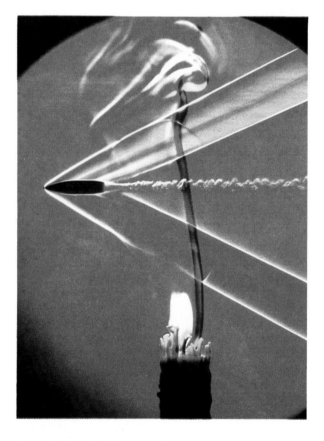

The technique of schlieren optics studies shock waves (in this instance those created by a bullet) by photographically recording their deflection of a beam of light. A special high-speed camera is used which has an electronic trigger connected to a microphone. The camera is set off when the shock wave reaches the microphone.

clear. Every car racing enthusiast knows the "mee-ee-eom" sound of a car approaching fast, then going away at the same speed. Yet if he were inside the car, he would hear that the engine note remains remarkably constant.

Distortion of Sound

As we have seen, sound travels at about 760 miles per hour (370 yards per second) at sea level. So when the racing car is standing on the starting grid, an observer in the grandstand hears a more or less steady note from its engine. But after the checkered flag is lowered, the car quickly achieves a substantial velocity. As it enters the homestretch, it may be traveling at 160 miles per hour (78 yards per second.) Thus the note of the engine is being thrown toward the observer at 78 plus 370 yards per second. This extra speed causes the sound waves from the steady engine tone to bunch up, increasing their frequency and with it the pitch. Only when the car is exactly in front of an observer will the true pitch be heard. As it races away, the sound waves are being slowed down by 78 yards every second, and so the sound waves are stretched out and the pitch is heard to drop.

This is a well-known effect—watch out for it in daily life — and is named after its describer, the nineteenth-century German physicist Johann Christian Doppler. (Incidentally, when the source of the sound travels so fast that its speed is greater than that of sound, a sonic boom results which is heard only at a distance from the source. This is a rather special case of the Doppler effect.)

We have seen earlier that the middle ear is equipped with a mechanism to prevent it from transmitting damagingly loud noises to the cochlea. This equipment requires a finite length of time

Johann Christian Doppler

Bunching and Stretching Sound Waves

A weak constitution often goes with a brilliant mind, and Johann Doppler was no exception. He was born in Salzburg, Austria, the son of a master stonemason, who planned a business career for him. But Johann wanted to be an academic, so when the astronomer Simon Stampfer, spotted his abilities and encouraged him to attend the Polytechnic Institute in Vienna, he willingly complied.

The precocious Doppler, finding the curriculum too one-sided, returned home after three years to study in private. From 1829–33, he taught mathematics at a school in Vienna and wrote his first papers in mathematics and electricity. However, his career came to a standstill, and he determined to emigrate. In 1835, en route to the USA, he journeyed to Munich, where he was unexpectedly offered a job teaching mathematics and accounting at the State Secondary School in Prague.

In 1841, Doppler became professor of elementary mathematics and practical geometry at the State Technical Academy in Prague. He was fascinated by a puzzling but commonplace phenomenon, which has become known as the Doppler effect: why does a sound, such as that of a train,

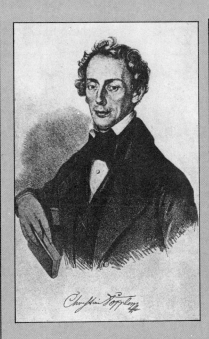

seem more highly pitched as the train approaches an observer and lower pitched when it recedes? Was it a trick of the ear or was there a change in the sound waves?

Within a year, Doppler proposed, and formulated mathematically, the principle that was to make his name immortal: the observed frequency of the sound wave is related to the motion of the source or, if the source is stationary, to the motion of the observer. Doppler explained this by saying that when a source moves, the waves in front of it "bunch together" and increase in frequency;

while those behind are "stretched out" and decrease in frequency. The extent depends on the velocity of the source.

To verify the Doppler principle, in 1845 some Dutch colleagues at Utrecht, led by C. H. D. Buys Ballot, organized what is probably one of the most extraordinary demonstrations in the history of science. They gathered together several trumpeters and several musicians who had perfect pitch. Seated in a railway truck, the trumpeters played various single notes as they were pulled back and forth by a locomotive. The musicians were stationed at a number of strategic points alongside the track where they identified the exact frequencies of the trumpet notes as the truck approached and receded. The experiment continued for two days and completely confirmed Doppler's principle.

Doppler died in Venice in 1853. The principle that bears his name has been modified by the relativity theorists of the twentieth century and is employed as a major tool in astrophysics. For example, it has accounted for the "red shift" phenomenon, which has led scientists to formulate the "big bang" theory of universal creation.

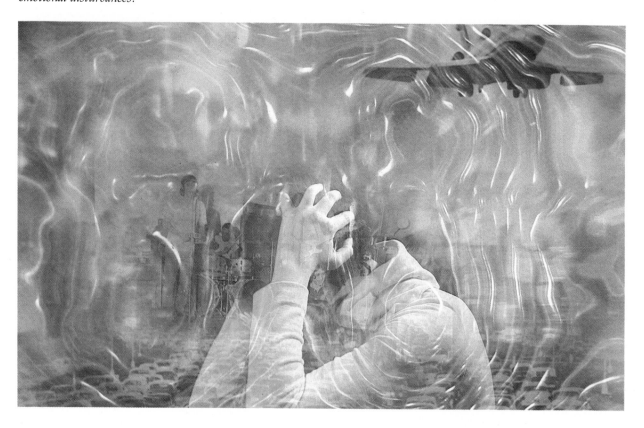

to be activated, and sudden, extremely loud noises, such as gunfire, may catch it unawares and result in partial or complete hearing loss for certain frequencies. But aside from this, the ear is well able to process differing sound intensities. The subjective loudness of a sound depends upon its intensity level above threshold, the duration of the sound and the width of the band of frequencies making up the sound (this is called the bandwidth), and it can be quantified in two ways.

First the test sound is matched against a reference sound — for example, a 1000 Hz continuous tone at fixed intensity — and the observer alters the intensity of the test sound until it equals that of the reference sound. This procedure is repeated for a wide range of frequencies, and the results averaged over a large number of subjects to produce an equal loudness contour. Each curve in the family of curves is said to have a loudness level, which is measured in phons; the number of phons is arbitrarily said to be equal to the sound pressure level (SPL), measured in decibels (dB SPL), of the reference tone of 1000 Hz. For example, a 60 Hz tone at 60 decibels is judged to have the same loudness as a 1000 Hz at 40 decibels, and is thus said to have a loudness level of 40 phons.

At high sound intensities, auditory sensation becomes uncomfortable. This discomfort threshold is called the loudness discomfort level and is — in round numbers — about 100 decibels. Louder noises cause actual pain and, above 140 decibels, may inflict damage on the middle ear. The 40 decibels equal loudness contour is used to calculate a measure of intensity that is used by environmental health authorities to decide when a sound level may be considered polluting. The measure is the total amount of noise, measured in decibels (dB SPL), passed by a filter with attenuation rates that match the 40 decibels equal loudness contour. One of the teasing problems of our time lies in deciding what sound levels constitute pollution; unfortunately, at levels below the discomfort threshold, there are, as yet, no nationally or internationally agreed standards.

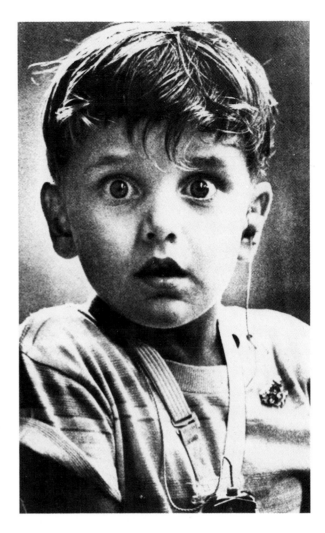

A five-year old boy shows his wide-eyed astonishment as he hears his own voice for the first time. With the aid of a special hearing aid, this deaf child is able to listen to a recording of his voice.

If people find themselves in a noisy environment, they may comment on it initially, but they soon get used to it: its loudness is perceived to decline. This happens fairly quickly at first and then progressively more slowly. In physiological terms, they are said to have "adapted" to the loudness, and measurement of the time course of loudness adaptation forms the basis for the tone decay test for various malfunctions of the cochlear nerve, as we shall see later. In normal ears, loudness adaptation is small — less than 15 decibels for one minute's exposure to a continuous tone produced at least 15 decibels above threshold for that frequency. How loudness adaptation occurs is not fully known, but it is thought to relate to the physiological adaptation of the firing rate of fibers in the cochlear nerve.

An extension of loudness adaptation occurs when we are subjected to levels of noise that are sufficiently high to reduce the sensitivity of our hearing via the middle ear reflex. Frequently sensitivity remains depressed after the stimulation has ceased, but most often, normal sensitivity soon returns. This is called temporary threshold shift, and, in severe conditions, it can last for days. Generally speaking, the magnitude of the shift increases with increases in intensity and duration of the stimulus, and the speed of recovery appears to depend upon the *total* energy of the stimulus (that is, stimulus intensity multiplied by its duration). For stimuli in excess of 100 decibels, the loss of sensitivity becomes rapidly more severe and may never fully return.

Damaging Effects of Noise

A person exposed to such stimuli may suffer a permanent threshold shift. In this context, it is interesting to note that loud, over-amplified rock music groups produce sound levels of around 140 decibels. By contrast, a symphony orchestra (not amplified) playing fortissimo (*fff*) produces about 90 decibels. Frequent attendance at rock concerts must damage hearing sensitivity.

The frequency at which the temporary threshold shift is maximal is close to the frequency of the high-intensity stimulus, or at least, the perceived frequency. At the highest intensities, the frequency at which the shift is maximal may be as much as half an octave or more above the fundamental of the high-intensity stimulus.

The sound environment is somewhat like an orchestra. Sounds rarely occur in isolation, and most stimuli occur close together or even simultaneously. If a single tone is presented to a subject at an intensity at or above its threshold, it will be perceived. But if a second tone of suitable intensity is presented simultaneously, the first tone may no longer be heard. Its intensity will now have to be increased before it is perceived. What has happened is that the second tone has masked the first. Generally the closer the frequency of the masking tone to that of the masked, and the greater its intensity, the greater will be the degree of masking.

Masking tones lower in frequency than those masked are more effective in masking than higher tones. Masking can still occur if the masking tone precedes that masked by up to 100 milliseconds, though generally the most effective masking occurs when both tones are presented simultaneously. Electrophysiological studies have shown that the

Sound Level (dB SPL)	Typical Example
180	Saturn rocket
140	Jet engine
	Loud rock group
	Threshold of pain
120	Damage to cochlear hair cells
110	Threshold for discomfort
100	Motor cycle engine Shouting at close range
90	Orchestra (fff)
80	Orchestra (ff) Busy street Shouting
60	Normal conversation Orchestra (mf)
50	Quiet conversation
30	Soft whisper Orchestra (ppp)
20	Country area at night
6.5	Mean threshold of sound at 1000 Hz

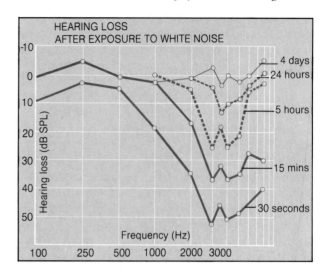

great majority of masking effects can be found in the neural response of the cochlear nerve, so the relation between the frequencies of the masking and masked tones are primarily determined by the nature of the response of the cochlear nerve.

Background, or "white," noise contains, by definition, all frequencies between certain limits at constant amplitude. In other words, the power spectrum of the white noise is flat. It has been calculated that the signal tone must be 5–15 decibels more intense than a background of white noise to be detected. This is why it is a strain to make yourself heard over a babble of voices producing a lot of power in the same frequency bandwidth in which you yourself are trying to project your signals.

Pinpointing Sound

You may have noticed that people deaf in one ear are able to process information about sound

frequency and intensity. But two ears are generally necessary to locate the position of a stimulus in the outside world. A sound emanating from one side of the head will strike one ear sooner than the other. As the speed of sound is constant, regardless of frequency, this "interaural" time difference will be the same at a particular location in space for any frequency. Delays of as little as 10 microseconds can be detected. Since the sound has to travel farther to reach the farther ear, it must excite more air molecules in its path than it had to in its journey to the nearer ear. Thus there will be a tiny intensity difference, which further aids location.

To pinpoint the source, the head is rotated until the interaural time difference and intensity difference are both nil. The sound source then lies straight ahead. Tests have been performed on blindfolded subjects to determine the minimum deviance in a sound source that can be detected. With a loudspeaker placed in front of a subject, a change in position of two degrees could be detected. But with the loudspeaker positioned at seventy-five degrees to one side of the head, the minimum change in position that could be detected was seven degrees. The angle was found to be smallest for low and relatively high frequencies and largest for middle and very high frequencies. Since we can locate a sound source accurately, even in a small room where sound is constantly reflected off walls, floor and ceiling, it has been suggested that the only cues we actually use are those associated with the

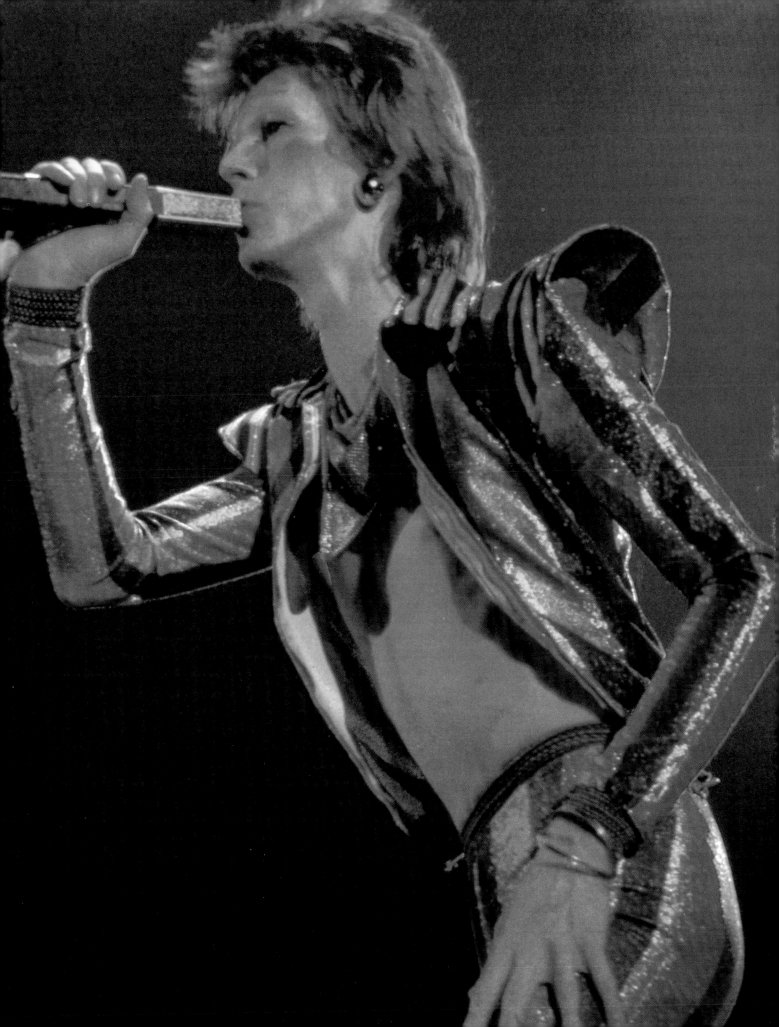

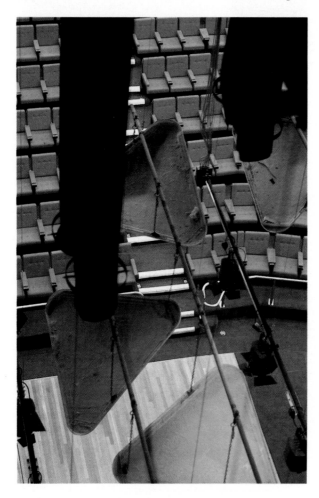

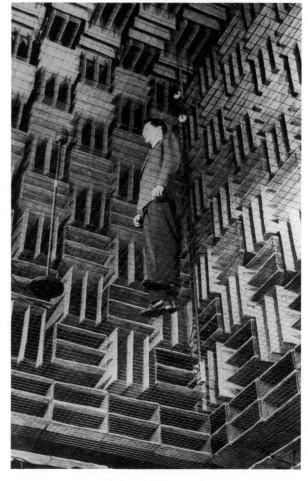

wavefront; somehow we can filter out those which are reflections.

An extremely difficult task is to locate sounds coming from above or below the plane of the ears. In a way not yet fully understood, the pinna plays an important role here. Incoming signals are transformed so that they are followed by a series of time-delayed replications. This effect occurs only for sounds in excess of 6000 Hz, for here the shortness of the waves interacts with the curls and grooves of the pinna. These structures provide a series of routes, each with its own time delays, for the sound to enter the meatus. In some way, the pattern of these delayed replications transmits the necessary information so that we instinctively look either up or down to find the source of the sound.

There is another phenomenon associated with two ears. At a noisy cocktail party, we may be able to converse quite happily with a friend even if the noise all around is quite loud. This is because we mentally locate the source of the sounds we are interested in and exclude all others. Visual contact also assists our localization of sound. But if we want to tune into another conversation nearby, we can do so without moving our heads. What we are doing is consciously bringing in some filters and no longer using others. The trick in this is to keep talking to our friends, while actually not hearing a word they are saying!

Understanding Speech

Human speech is an exceedingly complex train of frequencies, amplitudes, intensities and pulses of sound energy. The resolution of speech requires

Sonograms, or sound spectrums, give a picture of sound by plotting its frequency against the duration of the sound in seconds. (Frequency is the vertical axis.) Sonograms of the words "Hi" and "Tomato," spoken by both an American and an English woman, demonstrate certain differences in accent and style of speech. Note, for example, the high frequencies associated with the consonants in the word "tomato" in the English version, while in the American, the second "t" is all but dropped. More energy and emphasis is applied to the word "Hi" by the American speaker — hence its sharper and taller leading edge.

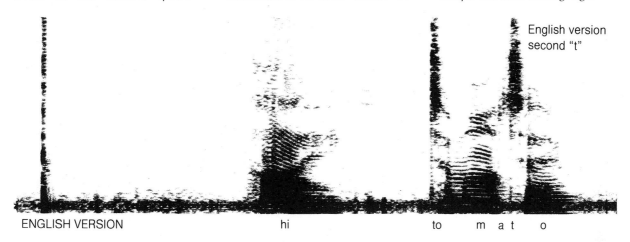

English version
second "t"

ENGLISH VERSION   hi   to   m   a   t   o

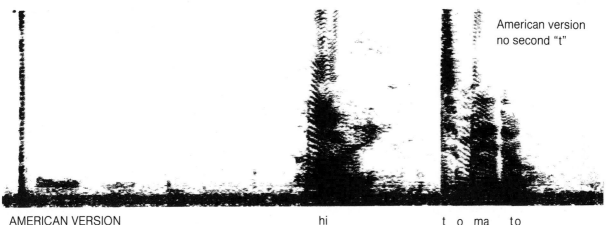

American version
no second "t"

AMERICAN VERSION   hi   t   o   ma   to

the resolution of multiple acoustic cues. For vowels, the relative spacing of harmonics or groups of harmonics is important; for diphthongs, the changes in frequency are also important. Consonants are characterized by broad waveband emissions and changes in the spacing of groups of harmonics. Generally speaking, we learn to recognize the juxtaposition of consonants and vowels in speech, and in each accent they are unique.

The same word or phrase in American and English accents may have a completely different structural appearance when analyzed on a sonogram. But it is a common experience that a few days' total immersion in the accent of another country or state resets our mental detection mechanisms.

Our mental ability does not stop there. If the first part of each word is clipped off — as often happens over satellite telephone links — we are actually able to assume that we have heard the whole word and can follow the conversation with little trouble. In fact, telephones are fascinating devices for anyone interested in how hearing happens. Telephones have the knack of filtering out the fundamental frequencies from the rises and falls in the voice's pitch, but since intonation is probably signaled by periodicity cues in the pattern of neuronal firings, the listener can fill in the missing elements.

So much for the normal, healthy ear. All too often, the ear falls prey to advancing years, and the associated hearing loss is probably one of the most common human complaints. Occasionally diseases and other malfunctions affect the ear, and these — and what can be done about them — form the substance of the next chapter.

51

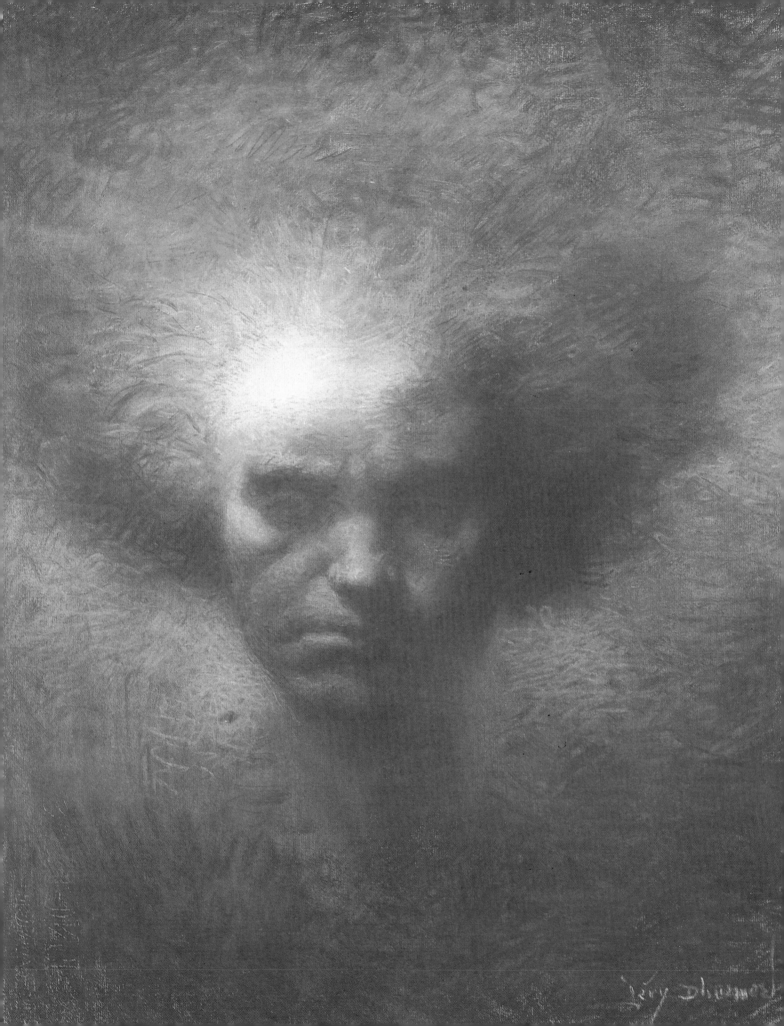

Chapter 3

The Imperfect Ear

Eight of ten people who read this book will experience trouble with their hearing. As we grow older, all our senses start to fail us, and, while more old people than young require eyeglasses to restore failing eyesight, impaired hearing is still perhaps the most common accompaniment to old age. A complex organ, the ear depends for perfect functioning upon a sequence of minute movements of the eardrum, or tympanum, the chain of little ossicles, the fluids in the cochlea and the basilar membrane. The resulting nerve impulses must then be processed by the brain into meaningful signals. Problems can start in any part of the ear, but let us work from the outside in.

The auditory meatus is seldom a significant source of trouble. Nobody really knows why earwax is produced, but the ceruminous glands that help produce wax are sometimes overactive and the meatus can become blocked. This wax blockage may be like a snowdrift, simply absorbing the sound and not allowing much to pass to the tympanum, or it may adhere to the tympanum. If the latter happens, the tympanum becomes too heavy to vibrate freely and requires higher than normal sound intensities to cause it to vibrate at all. A simple treatment is a dramatic and immediate remedy for both these complaints: the ears must be carefully syringed with warm soapy water to dislodge the wax.

The eardrum is sometimes a source of hearing troubles. A sudden blow to the ear can increase pressure in the auditory meatus and force the drum sharply inward. When this happens, the membrane may tear, resulting in the condition known as a perforated eardrum. A sudden, intense noise, for example a bomb explosion or nearby gunshots, can also rupture the eardrum. Small holes mend by themselves, usually within a few days, but healing can be hastened by a "splint" of cigarette paper placed by a physician over the torn edges.

A more serious disorder of the eardrum can occur

Much of the work of Lucien Lévy-Dhurmer (1865–1953) was inspired by the music of Beethoven, Debussy and Faure. In this portrait of Beethoven, Lévy-Dhurmer effectively conveys the feeling of isolation caused by deafness, the hazy, monochromatic style symbolizing the composer's blurred perception of sound. The painting succeeds in creating an impression of a man in a silent world.

53

The instinctive action of holding the hand to the ear when trying to hear, increases sound levels at the ear by about six decibels. More sound waves are trapped and more energy is available to the ear.

An illustration from the nineteenth-century medical book Family Physician *shows a patient having his ear syringed (below left). Syringing is still used today to dislodge wax from the ears.*

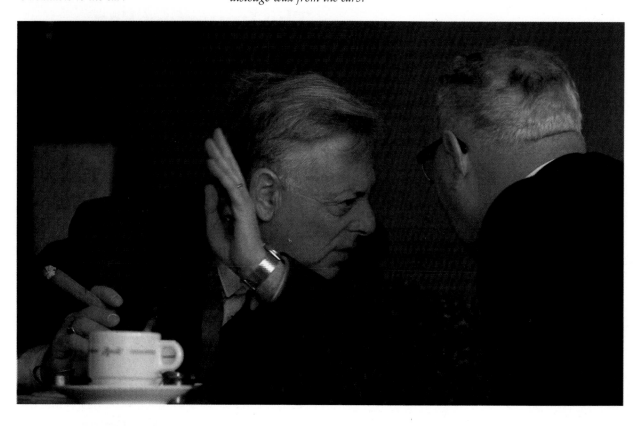

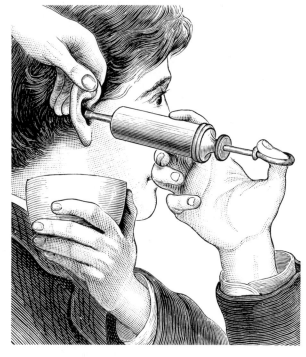

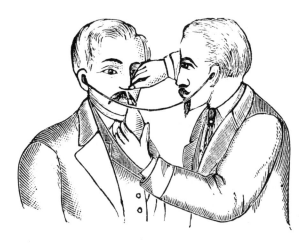

This nineteenth-century physician is examining the inner ear and Eustachian tube with an otoscope. Having pumped air into the tube, he listens to the resulting sounds in order to detect abnormalities.

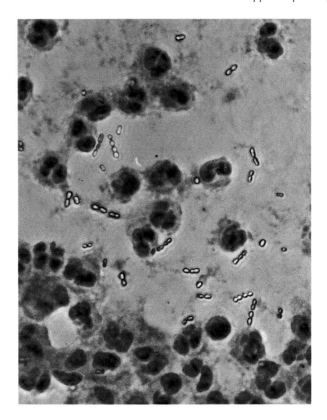

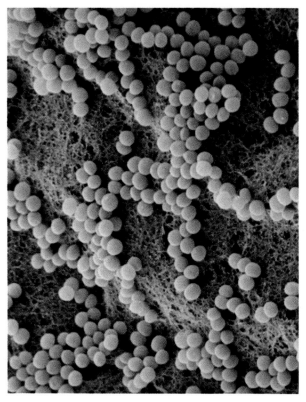

as a result of severe middle ear disease — otitis media — described below. The membrane becomes heavily scarred and loses some of its sensitivity. The only effective remedy is plastic surgery, in which part, or all, of the tympanum is replaced with a skin graft taken from the wall of the auditory meatus near the membrane. Such operations are usually highly successful.

The middle ear cavity is in direct and open contact with the back of the pharynx via the Eustachian tube, as we have already seen. The pharynx and upper respiratory tract are regularly besieged with bacterial and viral infections causing coughs, colds and sore throats — particularly in children — and the Eustachian tube can act as a kind of interstate highway, allowing microbes to reach the middle ear. If they do so, various types of middle ear infections (earache) result; doctors refer to these infections as otitis media, the chief causes of which are the streptococcus, pneumococcus and staphylococcus bacteria. If the delicate lining of the middle ear cavity is attacked by these bacteria, it swells and so

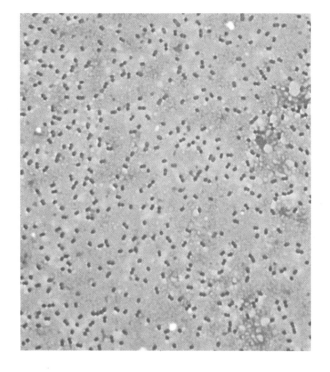

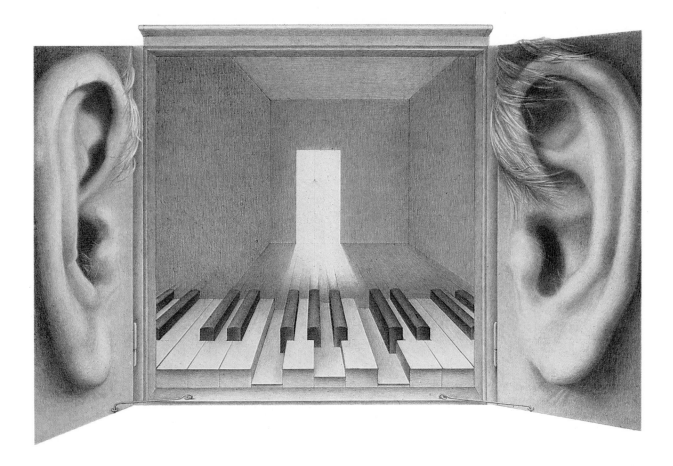

impedes the free movement of the hammer, anvil and stirrup — the ear ossicles. The resonance of the cavity, too, is affected, and the messages passed to the cochlea are distorted.

Nowadays middle ear infections are quickly eliminated by powerful antibiotic drugs, but, if the infection is particularly virulent and remains untreated, the tympanum may also become infected. There is much pain, and pus is discarded through tympanic perforations. The middle ear cavity is connected with a cavity in the mastoid bone — the bony protuberance just behind and below the ear, where the hangman places the knot of the noose. If severe, the infection may pass to this mastoid bone, causing mastoiditis, and from there even to the brain, resulting in the once-fatal meningitis. Early ear surgeons opened the mastoid bone to release the infectious pus and this operation was often successful. Such complications from otitis media are, thankfully, rare today.

Tinnitus, or ringing in the ears, can be caused by middle ear disease. These spontaneous, subjective noises can also result from lesions of the cochlea caused by excessive noise or by infection of the inner ear. High doses of aspirin are also known to

be associated with tinnitus. Generally, tinnitus causes no serious trouble except if the pitch of the noise masks the normal range of speech frequencies and impairs speech perception. The seat of the humming sensations appears to lie in the brain so there is no effective treatment. Bedřich Smetana, the great Czech composer, suffered from tinnitus for a few years before he became deaf at the age of fifty. The sound he heard was "the first inversion chord of A flat in the highest register of the piccolo." His genius was such that he was able to turn even the irritation of tinnitus to good effect, and he captured the sound in the first movement of his last quartet, *Arus meine leben* (*From my life*), composed in 1876.

Travel in unpressurized airplanes can trigger a minor malfunction of the auditory system. During ascent, the atmospheric pressure falls steadily and air in the middle ear is then at increasingly greater pressure than atmospheric. This pushes the tympanic membrane out slightly and restricts the vibrations of the ossicles. Until the Eustachian tube clears, allowing air to pass out of the middle ear, hearing is impaired. As the airplane descends, the reverse pressure changes occur and the eardrum

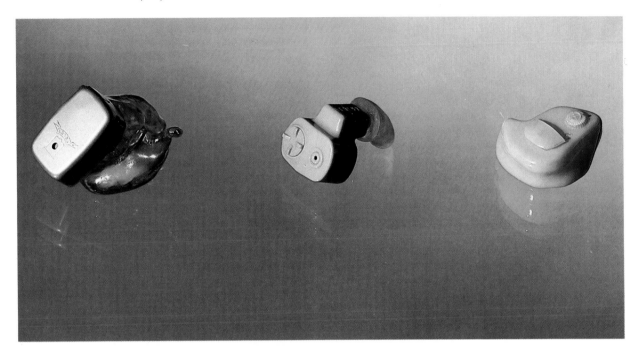

tends to be pushed in with the same effect on the ossicles. Air must be forced up the Eustachian tube by swallowing, or by exhaling with mouth and nose closed. Any infection of the Eustachian tube, possibly blocking the free flow of air, might cause the eardrums to rupture on ascent or descent. A blocked Eustachian tube can lead to trouble without the complication of air travel. As the air trapped in the middle ear cavity is absorbed by the tissues lining the cavity, the pressure decreases and forces the eardrum inward. The sufferer feels slightly deaf with a muffled feeling in the ears, but when the blockage in the tube clears, the complaint quickly disappears.

Loss of Hearing

The little ossicles themselves cause the most serious hearing problems. Their mobility decreases with age, resulting in what is called conductive hearing loss. Each ossicle is covered with a membrane and in otitis media this membrane may be affected, often influencing the articulation, or movement, points between the tiny bones. If these are permanently damaged, conductive hearing loss results, and sounds are attenuated, or made

quieter. The only remedy is to make sounds louder and in the past this was achieved with an ear trumpet, a kind of hunting horn, the narrow end of which was pushed into the meatus. The flared portion caught more sound energy than the unaided ear, and the whole structure was quite effective, if clumsy. Nowadays, with the help of microelectronics, hearing aids come in a variety of forms, many virtually unnoticeable in use.

For patients with severe articulation failure, a surgeon may perform an operation in which small slivers of skin and muscle are attached directly to the inside of the eardrum and to the stirrup. Thus the hammer and anvil bones are bypassed and sound is transmitted in a single step from eardrum to cochlea. (This arrangement is similar to the hearing system in reptiles, which have a single bone stretching from the eardrum to the cochlear window.) Although this rebuilt conductive mechanism lacks the control found in the normal ossicular system, it does offer partial restoration of hearing.

In a condition called otosclerosis, new filamentous bone grows over the stirrup, impeding its movement, and, if the new growth is severe, total deafness may result. One treatment involves

Glue ear, a condition in which sticky fluid collects in the ear, is common, particularly among young children. It is not known exactly why the condition occurs but it can be remedied surgically. Here a surgeon *operates to insert a grommet — a tiny plastic eyelet — in an opening he has made in the eardrum. This grommet must stay in place for a year or so; holding the eardrum open and allowing air into it in this way* *gradually disperses the fluid. Such delicate work as ear surgery has been made possible by the development of microsurgical equipment, which allows the surgeon to see clearly the minute structures of the ear.*

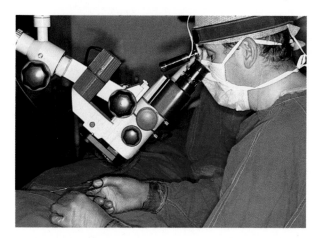

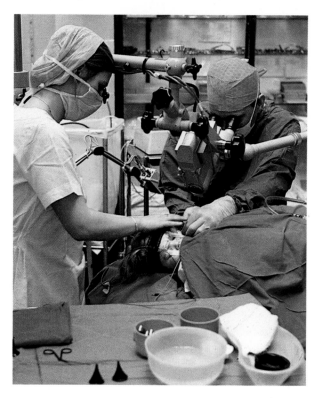

surgically making an opening into the cochlea, often via the horizontal semicircular canal. Called fenestration, from the Latin *fenestra*, meaning window, this operation requires the surgeon to destroy the ossicular chain before cutting a hole in the wall of the semicircular canal. The hole must be lined with a small flap of skin from the auditory meatus, and sound waves then pass through the air of the middle ear cavity directly from the eardrum. Reasonable hearing ability results, although occasionally the round window on the cochlea is also stimulated, and the patient hears no sound at all. Some patients also report suffering vertigo after this operation but generally agree that, despite these disadvantages, being able to hear something is preferable to deafness.

In the early 1950s, surgeons started to use a technique called stapes mobilization, in which the stirrup bone was physically manipulated in an attempt to free its footplate from fixation in the oval window. This most successful treatment restored the hearing of many patients to almost 100 percent. From this technique developed a delicate operation in which the bone-encrusted stirrup bone was removed (a stapedectomy), and a metal or plastic replacement inserted. This prosthesis was often a strand of metal with a small loop at one end to fix over the anvil and a larger loop at the other end to fit into the oval window of the cochlea.

Conductive hearing losses can be offset to some extent by sound traveling through the skull to the cochlea. In his last years, Ludwig von Beethoven suffered from severe otosclerosis and enhanced his failing hearing by propping a piece of wood between his mastoid bone and the piano. In this way he could still hear himself playing, since the sound bypassed his failing ossicles.

The cochlea and the auditory nerve are the most interior parts of the hearing system in which malfunction can occur. Damage leads to sensorineural hearing loss, for which, so far, there is no remedy. This condition can be caused in a number of ways but generally results from degeneration of the hair cells or the auditory nerve fibers. Hair cells, particularly those at the base of the cochlea in the region responsible for the perception of high frequencies, degenerate with age — from the age of about twenty we may lose about 1 Hz of our total perceptive range (about 20,000 Hz) every day, though for many people the rate of deterioration is slower. Long-term exposure to noise can, however, hasten degeneration of the cochlea and hair cells and such conditions used to be an occupational hazard of riveters, weavers and artillery men. Nowadays, an unfortunate side effect of some antibiotic drugs, such as dihydrostreptomycin and

Impossible for some people to contemplate, the view from a Manhattan skyscraper can induce a terrifying sensation of vertigo. This form of vertigo is psychosomatic and is caused by the effect of what the eye sees on the balance mechanism in the ear, bringing a feeling of dizziness. Vertigo can also result from those ear infections or malfunctions which disturb the balance mechanism, located in the inner ear.

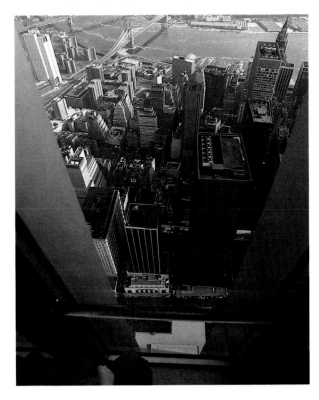

aminoglycoside, is cochlea damage, and diseases such as syphilis may reduce the blood supply to the cochlea, causing irreversible damage.

We do not yet know why cochlear damage leads first to a reduction in a patient's sensitivity to high frequencies. As we have said, the highest frequencies in human speech occur in the consonants, and patients with partial cochlear degeneration experience difficulty in perceiving speech, particularly in noisy surroundings.

Another little-understood condition is Ménière's syndrome. For unknown reasons, the pressure of the cochlear fluid rises, and the patient suffers tinnitus, hearing loss and vertigo — the latter causing giddiness, pallor and vomiting as experienced by poor sailors and fliers. The same symptoms can be caused by bacterial infection of the middle ear and, in some people, by looking down from tall buildings or cliffs. A new approach to cochlear malfunction, still in its research stage, is to bypass the cochlea altogether and to stimulate the auditory nerve directly. This operation has so far been performed primarily on animals under laboratory conditions, but results have been sufficiently impressive to encourage further work. A cochlear prosthesis is, however, still far from routine.

Occasionally a patient reports that he can no longer localize the point from which a sound emanates, or that he cannot distinguish changes in the duration of sounds. Such problems are always caused by damage to the auditory cortex in the brain's cerebral hemispheres, and are usually associated with incorrect comprehension of speech and errors in word order selection. As with many neural disorders, there is at present no remedy for this rare condition.

Such are some of the disorders that afflict our hearing system. But nowadays another problem gives real cause for concern — noise. As the world in which we live becomes increasingly noisy, noise is officially recognized by health authorities as a pollutant. The Industrial Revolution of the nineteenth century marked the start of the age of noise pollution. Steam engines drove spinning jennys and weaving looms, both incredible contrivances of clanking machinery. Everywhere noise filled the air, while money filled men's pockets. Amazingly, though, it took well over a hundred years for noise control legislation to benefit the ordinary worker. In the north of England for example, much of the equipment used by textile, spinning and weaving industries in the nineteenth century was still operating in the 1960s. An engineer working for a chain of movie theaters at this time noticed that amplifiers for the sound system were set to higher levels in the north of England than in the south. Constant exposure to the old machinery had reduced the average hearing sensitivity in that part of the country.

The Problem of Noise

Noise is undesirable for many reasons. Prolonged exposure to it results in partial deafness from hair-cell degeneration, while short-term exposure causes a temporary threshold shift. Noise can cause accidents by masking warning shouts and alarms. Sleep, concentration and so efficiency are affected by noise; it disrupts speech and social interaction and can be the cause of psychological problems ranging from bad temper to severe depression and even suicide.

Long-term exposure to loud noise results in hearing loss. After 20 years using noisy machinery such as nineteenth-century weaving looms (right), workers suffer decreased sensitivity in the frequency range of the sound made by the machinery. Prolonged exposure to such noise levels tends to destroy the hair cells in the inner ear — thus the loss of hearing sensitivity is permanent.

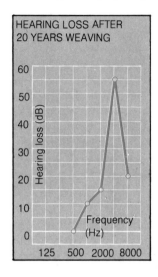

HEARING LOSS AFTER
20 YEARS WEAVING

Hearing loss (dB)

Frequency (Hz)

125   500 2000 8000

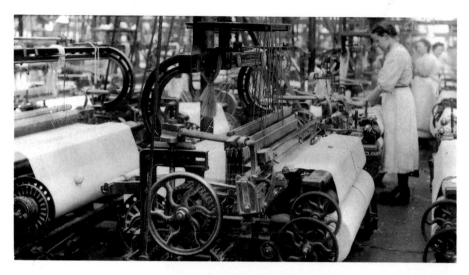

The U.S. Government has looked at the whole problem of noise pollution and has drawn up a table of permissible durations of exposure to various noise levels. For example, the permitted exposure to a noise level of 90 decibels is about 8 hours a day — traffic duty at a busy city intersection. With the help of such legislation, employers are becoming more aware of the problem of industrial noise, and great strides are being made in the reduction of noise at source. In the home and in leisure activities, however, levels of noise bombardment seem to increase. Tiny personal stereos — now so popular all over the world — have been used in Japan for over a decade, and their use is well correlated with a sharp rise in the rejection rate of trainee pilots for failure in critical hearing tests. Certainly, in most countries of the developed world, young people have diminished hearing abilities compared to previous generations. Only time will reveal what problems today's teenagers will experience when the normal hearing defects of old age make themselves felt on an already imperfect hearing system. (According to the U.S. figures, the. maximum exposure to a semiloud rock group should be only about fifteen minutes!)

More and more, doctors are recognizing that hearing malfunction tends to be accompanied by depression and a sense of isolation and insecurity. Sufferers feel that a major means of communication — and a specifically human one — has been lost to them. Social interaction is reduced and patients may become withdrawn, difficult to look after and even suicidal. Given this, and the fact that huge numbers of young people already have damaged hearing, it would seem crucial for governments everywhere to devote much more time and money to the treatment of the psychological correlates of impaired hearing.

Testing Hearing

Techniques for the investigation of hearing malfunction and disorders have been in use for many hundreds of years. The simplest employ tuning forks of the kind used by musicians to give a pure tone. In one nineteenth-century method, known as the Lateralization Test of Weber, a tuning fork was struck and pressed on the top of the head. In a normal subject, the sound is heard equally loudly in each ear. If the sound is heard more loudly in the patient's deaf ear, it indicates conductive hearing loss; if heard more loudly in the normal ear, it indicates sensorineural hearing loss. This test is simple, but unreliable. In another version, the tuning fork is first held near the pinna and then placed against the mastoid bone so that the sound is transmitted directly through to the cochlea. The duration of time for which a tone is heard provides a rough indication of the capability of the cochlea for perceiving that frequency. If the hearing is normal, the tuning fork will be heard for longer when presented to the pinna than when presented to the mastoid. But if the middle ear is diseased and the

William Hogarth's depiction of The
Enraged Musician *highlights the
disturbing aspects of unwanted
noise. The frustrated musician finds
concentration impossible as he battles
against the bombardment of sound*

*from beneath his window. All those
who live or work in a busy urban
environment will sympathize with
his predicament and appreciate the
tension, even fury, that can be
created by excessive noise.*

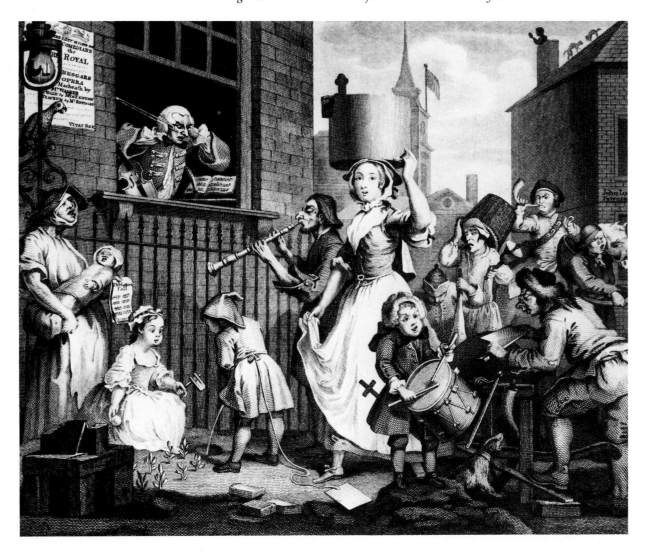

cochlea normal, the tone will be heard for longer when applied to the mastoid. This test is still used by some hearing specialists although tuning forks have given way to electronic tones.

The audiometer, a device that produces pure tones at varying intensities, is used by most hearing specialists in their tests. The patient is asked to indicate the least intensity at which he or she can hear a particular tone so that a frequency threshold curve can be drawn for comparison with the norm. Such an instrument is able to indicate only that malfunction occurs; it cannot say in which part of the ear the malfunction lies. To test whether the trouble lies in the middle ear, an impedance audiometer may be used. A plug is fitted into the patient's ear, and a small pressure generated into the auditory meatus. A tone is then presented to the ear, and the minute pressure changes in the auditory meatus measured. If the tympanum, chain of ossicles and oval window are all functioning normally, a specific pattern of pressure change should be observed. If there is middle ear damage, the pattern will be different, and further investigation of that area is indicated.

The human ear is an amazing instrument of the most extreme precision. It allows us to communicate via the complex medium of speech, and from this has developed the universal love of

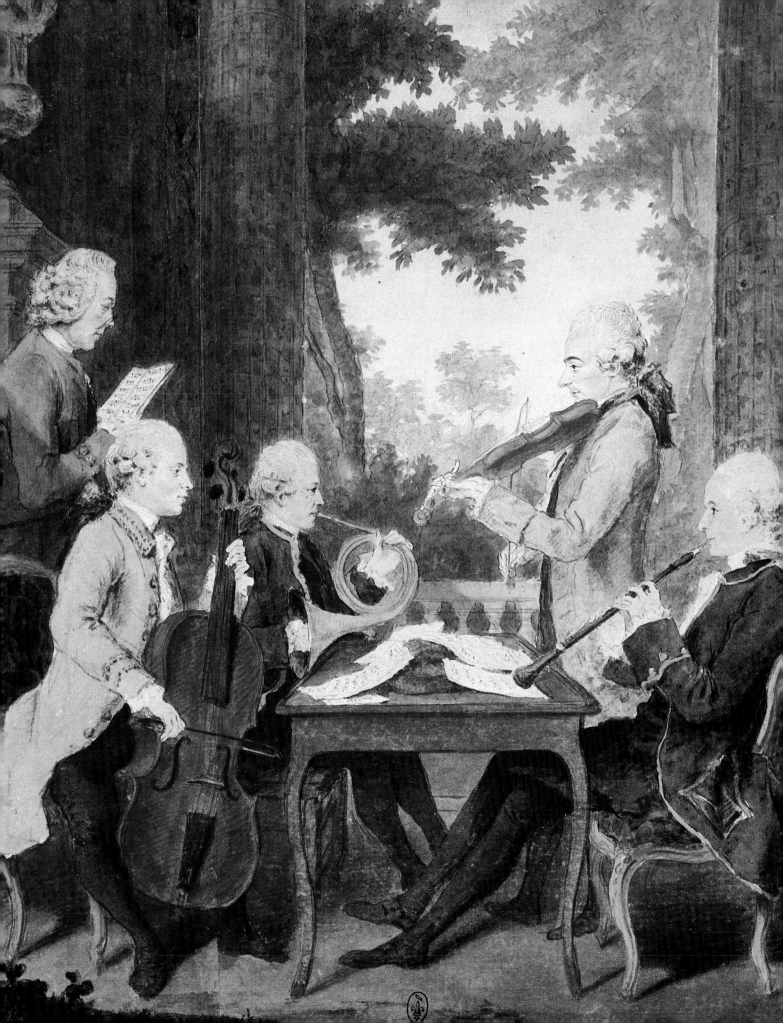

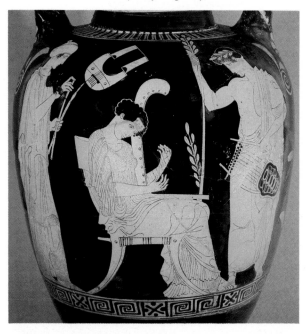

humans for music. The appreciation of music requires an auditory system capable of accurate discrimination of frequency. But the human ear, when coupled to the human brain, is far more than just a straightforward discriminatory machine. Music is able to influence human mood in an extraordinarily subtle manner. The great composer Handel regarded any key signature with five, six, seven and eight sharps in it as being associated with Heaven — the so-called transcendental keys. He reserved G minor for a sense of urgency and jealousy, and E minor for the creation of an elegaic mood. Bright daylight, sunshine and green pastures are suggested by strident music in G major, gloom and despondency by F minor. Western music is based on the scales established by the Greeks, who were the first to associate different emotions with different modes of the scales to which they gave names. The Dorian mode was said to be manly, courageous and dignified, while the Lydian mode was supposed to induce softness and self-indulgence and was thought to share with the Ionian mode a certain voluptuousness.

All of these modes can be played on a piano by any half-competent musician; there is no difference between them except for the intervals, or jumps, between the main stepping stones from octave to octave. With its ability to discriminate pitch, the human ear can transmit complex signals to the brain that cause even more complex changes in mood.

Now try this. Once the day's work is over and preparations for the evening meal are under way, put your favorite music on the stereo and relax. Feel your mood change as the music soothes you. Delicious aromas of cooking food waft from the kitchen and your mouth starts to water. While your highly sophisticated ear is changing your outlook on life, your more earthy senses of taste and smell remind you that you have to eat. But are these latter senses so earthy? The following chapters may cause you to reevaluate this view of the "chemical" senses.

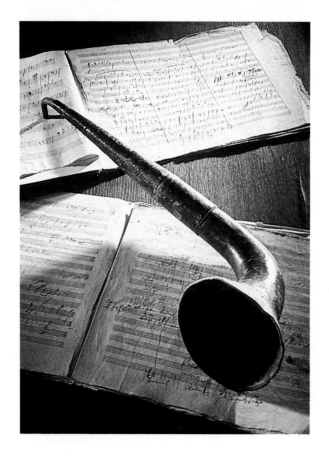

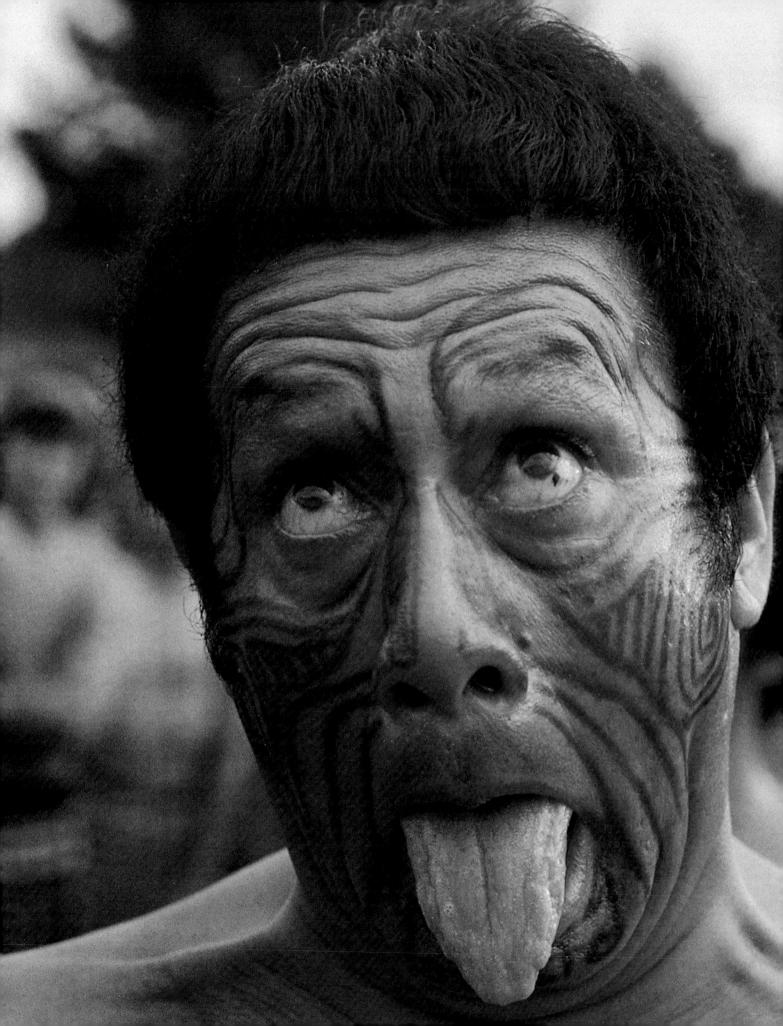

Chapter 4

The Versatile Tongue

An extraordinary quirk of biology links the ear with the tongue. The chorda tympani nerve, a branch of the VIIth cranial nerve, passes through the middle ear, and one of its several destinations is a portion of the brain that receives gustatory sensory information from the tongue's taste buds. The nerves carrying the nerve impulses saying "fresh celery taste" actually pass through the chain of ear ossicles, which are busy generating parallel auditory nerve impulses about the crunching sound of chewed celery. Other links between the ear and the tongue are more profound, however, not least that between the tongue, modulator of speech, and the ear, decoder of speech.

Many human organs are multifunctional. The pancreas, for example, produces a potent concoction of digestive enzymes, including trypsin for the breakdown of food macromolecules, but it is also the synthesizer of the crucial blood-glucose-controlling hormone, insulin. The liver elaborates bile constituents and holds massive reserves of glycogen but is also the main detoxifying organ in the body. Such adaptiveness is a consequence of the economy and efficiency that result from the molding forces of natural selection. The tongue is a particularly splendid example of an "organ for all functions." Although people are rarely conscious of the workings of the tongue, here is a part of the body with an extraordinary diversity of facilities.

Used in chewing, sucking and swallowing, the tongue is, at the same time, the preeminent organ of taste. It also has another vital function as one of the principal modulators in the complex physical mechanisms that produce speech — the most consciously structured and elaborate of our modes of communication with other human beings. The versatile tongue is, therefore, both the location of one extremely sensitive sensory ability (taste) and the producer of the stimuli that excite another sense with enormous social significance (hearing).

Sticking the tongue right out is a traditional gesture of greeting for the Maori tribespeople of New Zealand. Used in dances, the expression is initially intended to frighten off potential enemies. Once friendship is established between the participants, however, they end the dance by again sticking out their tongues, this time as a sign of peace.

65

A vertical section of the human tongue magnified about 100 times shows the multilayered mucous membrane (top left). Beneath the membrane are muscle fibers, which make up much of the tongue's bulk.

A magnified view of the surface of the human tongue shows light-topped filiform papillae and a scattering of red-topped fungiform papillae. The median furrow runs across the picture.

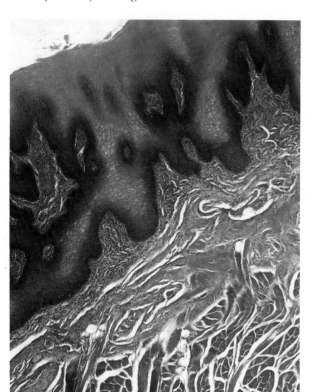

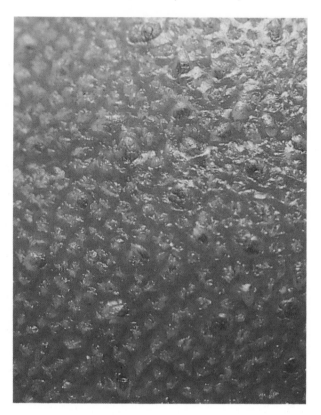

The tongue is a predominantly muscular organ, which, as a result of the differential contraction of the striated, voluntary muscles within it, has an immense capacity for both slow and rapid shape changes. It is made up of the following components: a network of bundles of striated muscle fibers, fibrous tissue, fat and lymphoid masses, mucus-producing glands and a covering of mucous membrane.

Muscles make up the bulk of the tongue's volume. They are arrayed in two complex sets, both of which have laterally paired muscle blocks so that the left and right halves of the tongue have their own independent musculature. The two halves are divided internally by a fibrous median septum. The only external evidence of this compartmentalization is the median furrow, a visible groove on the surface of the tongue. It is the diversity of these muscle arrays and the intricacy of their interaction that ensures the flexibility of the human tongue and the delicacy and multiplicity of its shape changes. Something of the structure can be understood by

examining a slice of ox tongue. While most meat has an obvious muscle fiber orientation, tongue has muscles going in all directions.

Each lateral set of glossal, or tongue, muscles consists of two arrays: one of intrinsic muscles, which do not leave the tongue, and one of extrinsic muscles, which run from the bulk of the tongue itself to the bony prominences surrounding it. Apparently free in the floor of the mouth, the tongue is, in fact, anchored in all directions to bones — to the lower jaw in front, the hyoid bone below, the base of the skull behind and the palate above. Each of the four muscle blocks on each side accomplishes particular gross movements of the tongue. The genio-glossus runs from the inner surface of the front of the lower jaw into the tongue from tip to base. When the two genio-glossals are contracted at the same time, the tongue is protruded by its whole foundation being pulled forward. The second type of extrinsic muscle is the hyo-glossus — a flat strap of muscle that passes from the side of the tongue onto one arm of the wishbone-shaped hyoid

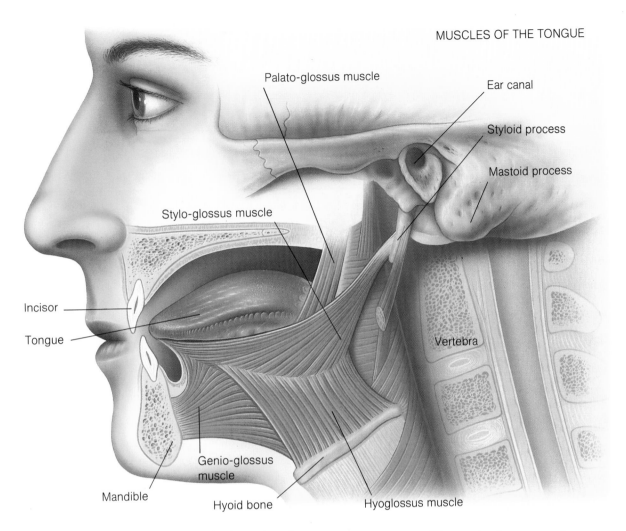

Palato-glossus muscle

Ear canal

Styloid process

Mastoid process

Stylo-glossus muscle

Incisor

Tongue

Vertebra

Genio-glossus muscle

Mandible

Hyoid bone

Hyoglossus muscle

bone in the throat. Contraction of the hyo-glossals pulls down the sides of the tongue. Third are the stylo-glossals, which link the sides of the tongue to the base of the skull via the bony styloid processes, extending downward from the temporal bones. Contraction of these muscles pulls the tongue back and upward. The fourth of these muscle sets are the palato-glossals that connect the sides and upper region of the tongue to the rear of the palate and are able to lift the sides of the tongue.

Just as the combined and integrated activities of the extrinsic muscles of the eye make the eyeball point with precision in any direction, so too can the externally linked muscles of the tongue generate movements of almost any type. These bulk movements, however, are relatively gross, and it is the intrinsic glossal muscles that provide the ability for detailed shape changes of considerable three-dimensional exactness. The fibers of the intrinsic muscles are grouped into four assemblages: two running from the front to the back of the tongue, one transversely and the last vertically.

The muscles that connect the tongue to the bones around it — the extrinsic muscles — take up a surprisingly large space within the arc of the lower jaw. A cutaway diagram of the left side of the face shows the four sets of extrinsic muscles on this side of the head. A similar group of four muscle sets lies on the right side of the head. Both groups work together in a coordinated way to bring about gross movements of the tongue. Within the tongue, there are further, intrinsic muscles, which control the detailed shape changes of the organ.

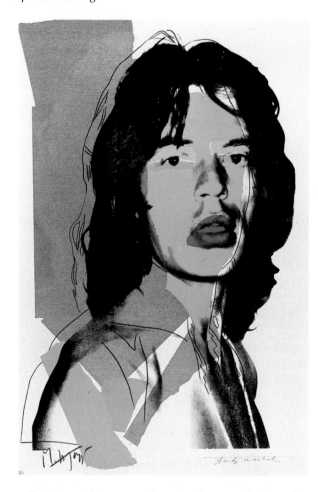

there are some general patterns of activity. The whole tongue may be moved up or down in the mouth cavity, thereby altering the size of the air passageway and its resonating properties. At the same time, the free tip of the tongue can quickly be applied to any region of the palate, inner surfaces of the teeth or lips; while the rear parts of the tongue body can touch to the walls of the buccal cavity and pharynx. These activities of the tongue induce checks in the pattern of outward-moving air and are at the heart of the mechanisms for several consonant sounds. The "ke" consonant sound, for instance, results from an expiration block in the posterior tongue region, while the application of the free tongue tip to the tips of the upper incisor teeth produces the "th" sound.

Functions of the Tongue

This mechanistic analysis of the muscular activity associated with the process of human speech may seem a simplistic, crude approach to the wonderful richness and profundity of this mode of expression. A mother's lullaby, a passionate duet from *Fidelio*, the persuasive cadences of a political orator, all are built from the same underlying simple pattern. Out of the human mind and the coordinated contractions of eight plus four muscle sets, we make sounds that inspire love, envy, respect — indeed any human emotion. Those same sounds can transmit precise information from one person to another with tremendous speed and remarkably high fidelity.

Asked to list the functions of the tongue in order of importance, many people might find it hard to decide whether taste or speech should top their list. Although most of us would find it immeasurably harder to lead a normal life without the power of speech than without the faculty of gustation, many instinctively feel that life without taste would be a dramatically diminished existence. The surface topography of the tongue is as fascinating as its internal musculature. Here, at the interface between the outside world and the tongue, are the array of receptor cells that signal information about the chemical composition of material in the mouth to the brain — the first and most vital step in the perception of taste.

The sense of taste, like smell, has little occupied the minds of scientists, both ancient and modern.

In a conscious, nonsleeping human being, the tongue is in almost continuous activity, and during any vocalization it is constantly moved from its rest position. At rest, the tongue, with a convex upper surface over its front two-thirds, fits neatly into the roof of the closed mouth. The origins of the air vibrations from which speech is constructed are, of course, the corresponding sets of vibrations set up in the vocal cords within the larynx during expiration. The actual phonemes of speech, however, result from modifications of the basic vocal-cord-produced sounds by temporary alterations in the configurations of the spaces in the head through which these sounds must pass.

Together with the lips, the tongue plays a central role in engendering these all-important modifications. The precise movements and shape changes of the tongue differ for each individual sound, but

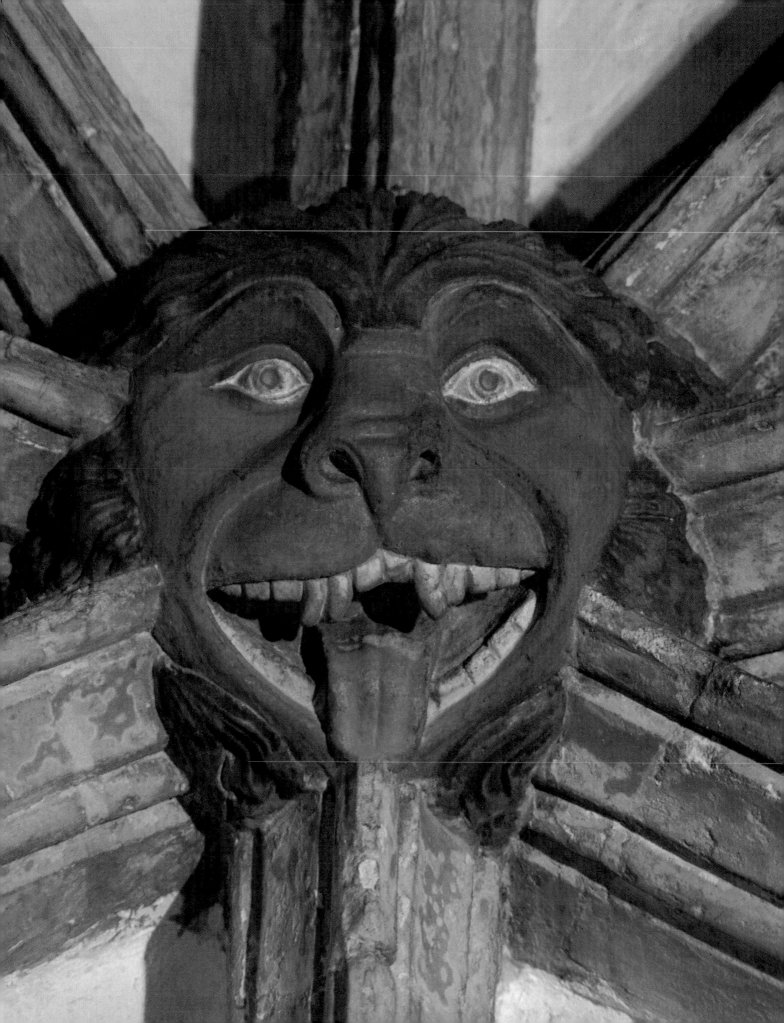

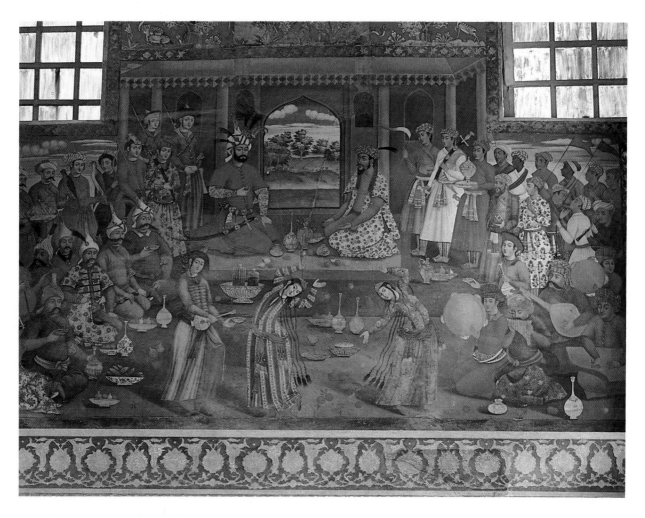

Anaxagoras of Clazomenae (500–428 B.C.) believed that like things could not be affected by like, thus taste must be produced by the meeting of opposites. Sweetness would be sensed by virtue of the sourness with which man is born, rather than by means of itself. A theory suggested by Democritus of Abdera (460–360 B.C.), was that sensations of taste arose directly from atoms of a certain shape that fitted exactly into receptacles on the tongue. The Roman poet Lucretius (c.90–55 B.C.) expressed this more lyrically, saying that the particles of sweetness were smooth and caressed the pores of the palate, while sour and bitter particles had barbed edges and treated the pores roughly.

Aristotle of Stagira (384–322 B.C.) believed taste to be a kind of touch and, since food is something the tongue can touch, that taste was the sense of nutrition. He noticed how water, passed through other substances, became "charged" with certain qualities, which conveyed the sensation of flavors. Taste arose when these qualities were transferred to the moist tongue. From there they were carried via the blood to the heart — then thought to be the seat of all sensations, the seat of the soul.

Although Galen of Pergamum (A.D. 131–201) said far less about taste than the other senses, he did correctly identify one of the nerves responsible for relaying the sensations of taste to the brain. This nerve is now called the glosso-pharyngeal nerve (cranial nerve IX). He also proved conclusively that all sensations are perceived in the brain, not, as Aristotle had thought, in the heart. To Galen, the organ of taste was "moist and like a sponge," stimulated by elementary particles and coarse corpuscles. His theory was that moisture was extracted from the humors of the blood by the salivary gland and provided a fluid in which to suspend the particles and corpuscles and enable them to contact the tongue sufficiently closely to generate sensations of taste.

Little progress in the study of taste was made until the invention of the microscope allowed scientists to take a close look at the tongue. In the seventeenth century, Marcello Malpighi (1628–94), an Italian who was one of the greatest of the early microscopists and the founder of histology,

70

realized that the papillae on the tongue were the organs of taste. Two centuries later, in 1867, Gustav Schwalbe and C. Löwen, German scientists working independently, described how certain tiny structures embedded in and around the papillae appeared to be the actual mediators of taste. Löwen named them taste buds and Schwalbe suggested that there may be as many as 400 of these structures in each papilla.

The Surface of the Tongue

Although twentieth-century technology can reveal the structure of the taste bud in almost molecular detail, there is still some doubt about its exact method of functioning, as we shall see later. Look at your own tongue in a mirror; there is no better way of understanding the surface complexity packed into this fascinating organ. With tongue protruded, only the front two-thirds are really visible. This is the so-called palatine section. Behind it, and separated from the front by a transverse groove, is the pharyngeal section. A minimum of tongue maneuvering quickly demonstrates that the upper and lower surfaces are different in character. The underside is covered with smooth mucous membrane, which is thin and loosely connected to the underlying muscles. This smooth expanse is broken in the midline by a fold of tissue, the frenulum linguae. In babies and young children, this fold is sometimes too extensively attached to the tongue and mouth floor, resulting in a relatively tethered tongue, or "tongue-tied" condition. This is easily reversed by minor surgery.

The upper surface of the tongue is much more complicated. The palatine section is completely covered with closely packed, short projections, or papillae. These give the upper surface of the front of the tongue its rough, velvety appearance. Behind the transverse groove, in the posterior pharyngeal zone, the surface changes to a series of low rounded "hillocks," difficult to see in one's own mouth without the aid of a second small mirror. These knobbly bulges are caused by underlying lymphoid nodules, like tiny tonsils, and clusters of mucus-producing glands like those mixed up with the muscle strands at the tip of the tongue. If the posterior bulges are in view, it should also be possible to see a central depression in the tongue

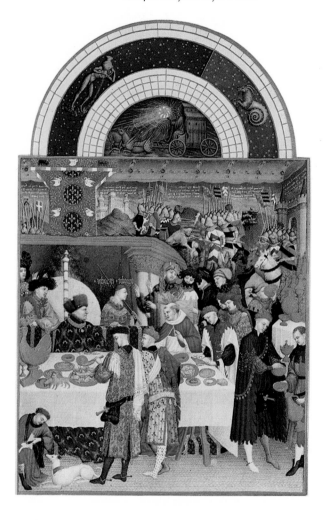

surface, just behind the transverse groove. This umbilicuslike cavity has a remarkable embryological history. It indicates the site where, early in intrauterine development, part of the floor of the human embryo's mouth invaginates, or indents, to provide cells for the construction of the primitive thyroid gland. This developmental event is effectively completed nineteen days after conception, and, for a while, the embryonic thyroid gland is connected via a tube with the floor of the mouth. The tube later solidifies, and the depression is all that remains at the surface to show where this crucial endocrine gland had its fetal beginnings.

The papillae on the tongue's upper surface carry by far the largest concentrations of taste buds of any portion of the mouth's inner lining. Taste buds are

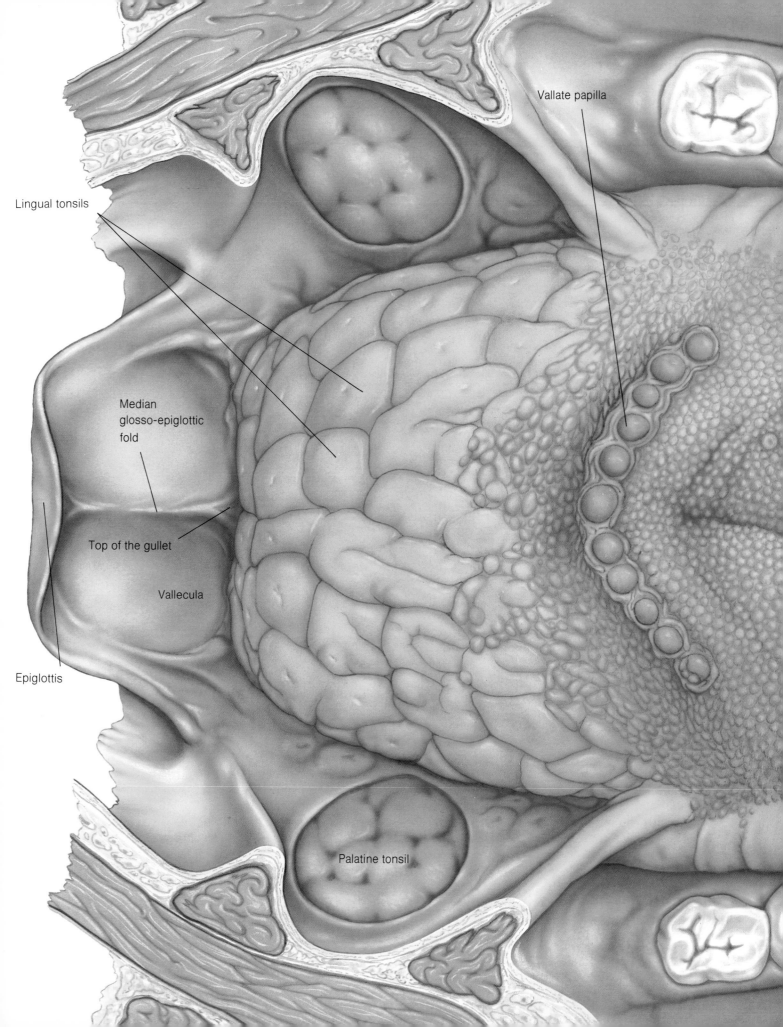

Vallate papilla

Lingual tonsils

Median
glosso-epiglottic
fold

Top of the gullet

Vallecula

Epiglottis

Palatine tonsil

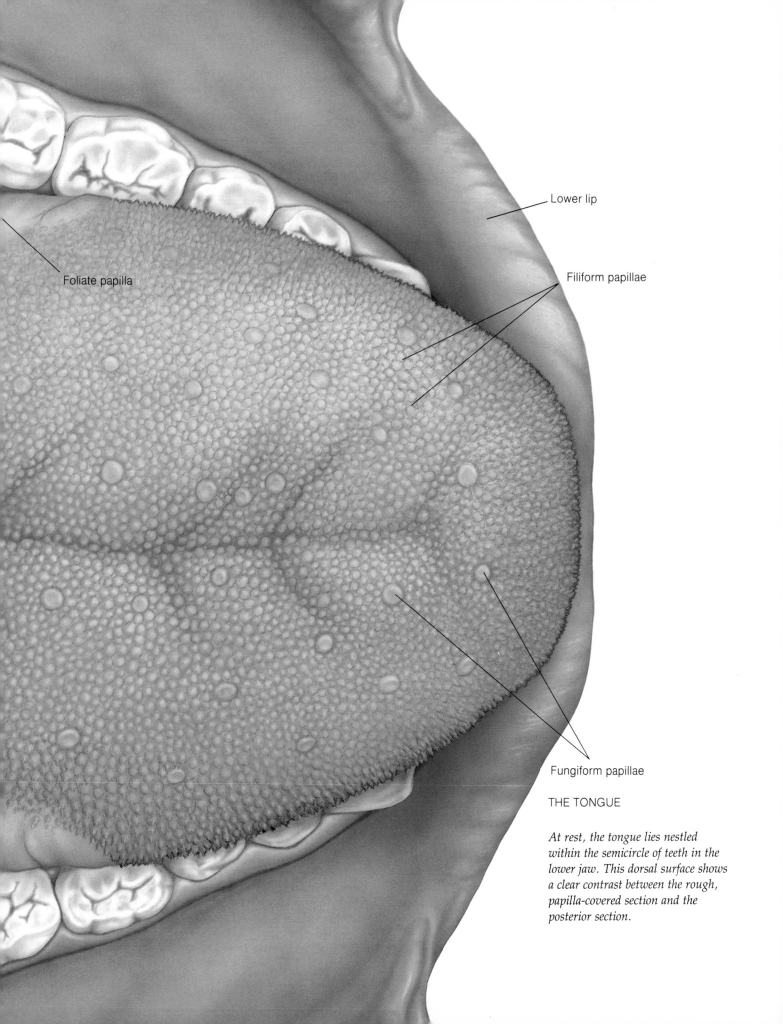

Lower lip

Filiform papillae

Foliate papilla

Fungiform papillae

THE TONGUE

At rest, the tongue lies nestled within the semicircle of teeth in the lower jaw. This dorsal surface shows a clear contrast between the rough, papilla-covered section and the posterior section.

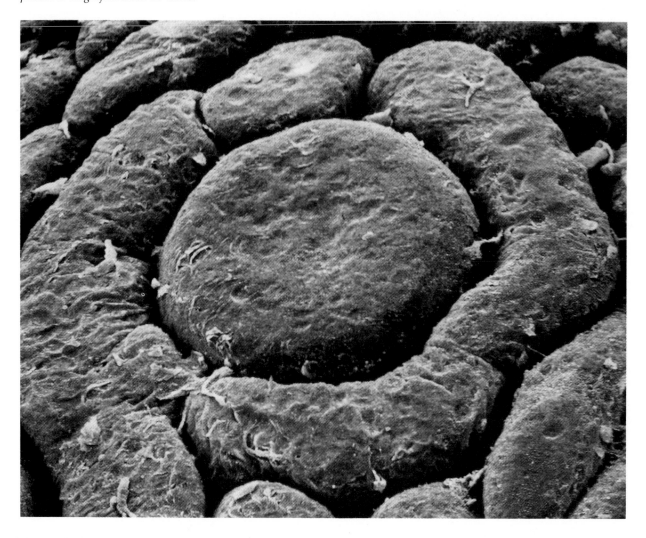

the microscopic clusters of sensory cells that are directly responsible for gustatory chemoreception in the mouth. They are not confined to the tongue; a thinner scattering of them is to be found in many parts of the mouth's mucous membrane, including the epiglottis, pharynx, larynx, soft palate and uvula. There are also taste buds on the mucous membrane of the upper third of the esophagus, allowing us still to taste food as it is being swallowed. The glossal papillae, though, are the most important location for taste buds.

Inspection of the dense pile of papillae that decorates the upper surface of the tongue reveals that the projections come in several shapes and dimensions; some are rare, others extremely numerous. The papillae types have been categorized in a number of different ways, but one of the more widely accepted classifications splits them into four basic variants: filiform, foliate, fungiform and vallate papillae.

Types of Tongue Papillae

Filiform papillae, sometimes referred to as conical papillae, are the most numerous type. Most are arranged in fairly regular rows, parallel to the median longitudinal groove of the tongue. At the free tip, the rows run across the tongue. Some of these papillae are simply conical, while others have frilled tips, with each branch of the peak itself being roughly conical. The epithelial coat of the filiform papilla follows all the tongue's surface irregularities, and its outer cell layers are continuously and progressively converted into dead, fairly hard "scales." The white-coated tongue, which sometimes accompanies disease processes not specifically to do with the mouth, is partly due to the accumulation of these scales in excessive numbers. The coat also contains free white blood cells.

Although the filiforms are the most numerous of the human tongue papillae, microanatomical evidence shows that they are not involved in the perception of taste. Their mucous membrane does not appear to carry any taste buds whatever. Filiform papillae have a more mechanical function, like the teeth on a file, hence their shape and their surface-hardened construction. The tongue's cleansing lick is effected by the abrasive qualities of the filiform papillae, followed up by the antibacterial properties of the applied saliva, which contains potent bacteriocidal substances, such as lysozyme. Members of the cat family have specialized, spine-shaped filiform papillae, with backward-facing points, which turn their tongues into highly efficient rasping devices. They use their tongues for scraping off the surface of fresh meat when feeding and for grooming their fur. Our filiform papillae are less specialized but may be said to carry out the same types of activity.

The remaining three types of tongue papillae all have taste buds on their surfaces and are concerned with the sense of taste. The numbers and locations of these gustatory papillae are highly ordered and differ from species to species. The various great apes, for example, show considerable differences in their papillae.

The human complement of gustatory papillae includes from seven to twelve vallate (sometimes called circumvallate) papillae. These, the largest of the tongue's papillae, are arranged on the upper surface in a distinctive pattern: a V-shaped formation of bulges directed toward the throat. More numerous than the vallates are the fungiform papillae, which are particularly prominent at the tip of the tongue and along its lateral edges. Finally, the foliate papillae, also referred to collectively as the lateral organs, are clustered into two groups, one on each side of the tongue, positioned just in front of the "V" of the vallate papillae.

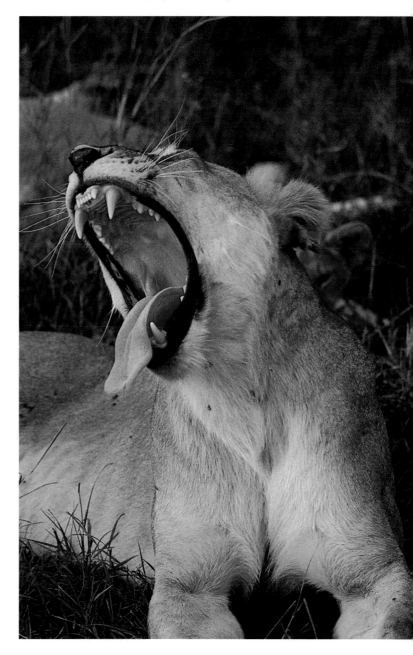

On the sides of the central papilla visible in this photomicrograph of a mammalian tongue, seven taste buds (light oval structures) can be seen. The apical pores of the taste buds are directed outward.

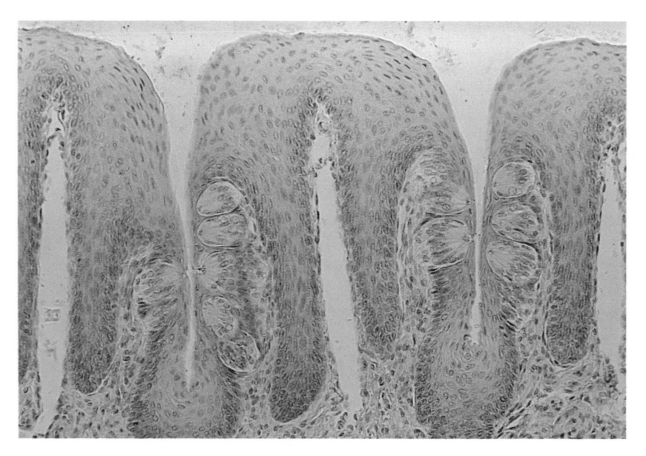

The differing structure of the three types of taste papillae and their characteristic positions on the tongue have led a number of workers in the field to conclude that each papilla type responds selectively to a particular taste quality. Most modern findings, however, suggest that this is an overly simplistic analysis and that the structural basis of taste discrimination must be sought at a different, probably molecular, level of receptor organization. We shall return to this evidence in the next chapter.

The architecture of a vallate papilla is rather complex, with the taste buds in it being distributed over a convoluted, three-dimensional surface. Perhaps the best analogy for the vallate's structural framework is a round, domed castle keep, surrounded by a deep moat, itself protected by a steep-sided dike. Large numbers of taste buds are disposed in tiers on the outer walls of the "keep" and on both inner and outer banks of the "dike." At the bottom of the "moat" are secretory gland cells, which

produce a watery mucus — the immediate external environment of the taste buds.

Detailed microanatomical studies of the human tongue carried out during the 1930s produced some fascinating statistics about the natural history of the taste buds in our vallate papillae. During childhood and adulthood up to the age of seventy, each of the seven to twelve vallate papillae bears from 250 to 270 taste buds. Later in life — between the ages of seventy-four and eighty-five — the density of vallate taste buds drops significantly to less than 50 percent of the normal adult total. The aging process damages our powers of taste just as it does so many of our other faculties.

The structure of individual fungiform and foliate papillae is simpler than that of the vallate type. A fungiform papilla is somewhat similar to the central region of a vallate, with an almost spherical shape, a flattened top and a narrowed base connecting it to the underlying tissues. The name fungiform

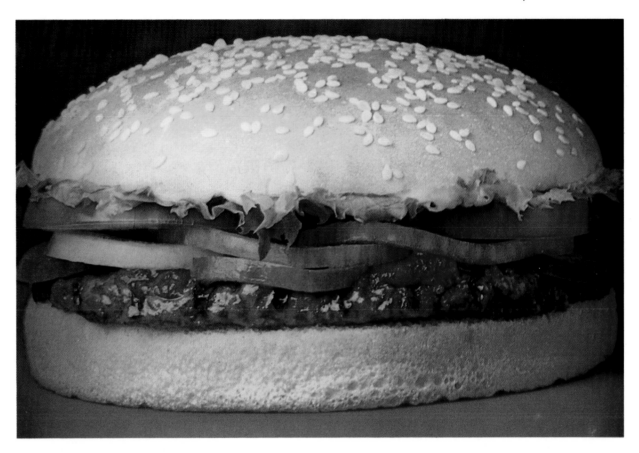

A simple hamburger in a sesame seed bun is good to eat, but the addition of onion, tomato and lettuce and the sweet-and-sour taste of catsup gives a more complex taste, adding zest and interest to a plain meal.

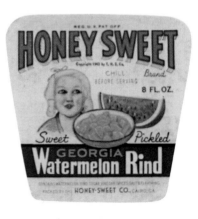

All four types of taste — sweet, sour, salt and bitter — are contained in this jar of pickle. An easy way of enlivening a meal, pickle also stimulates the gastric juices and aids digestion.

(fungus-shaped) is an appropriate one: the scattered fungiforms looking like a crop of miniscule, if somewhat globular, mushrooms popping up through the surrounding herbiage of filiform papillae. The foliates, too, are aptly named. Foliate means leaflike, and each of these papillae is an elongate fold, resembling a leaf seen edgeon. Taste buds are scattered over the epithelium of the fungiforms and on the opposed walls of the adjacent foliate papillae.

The Sensory Taste Buds

In considering the structure and arrangement of the taste papillae on the tongue, it has so far been tacitly assumed that a papilla carrying taste buds serves a sensory role in relation to taste. Although the connection is so confidently referred to in everyday life — advertisements promise that a certain dish will "tickle the taste buds" — the reality of these sensory entities continues to perplex investigators to

Carl Pfaffmann

Electrophysiologist of Taste

Early in his career, Carl Pfaffmann began to concentrate on the physiology and psychology of the chemical senses, particularly taste. Searching to clarify the relationships between behavior, perception and the mechanism of chemoreception, he quickly found this to be no easy task; no one physiological mechanism could account for any one psychological process.

Born in 1913, in Brooklyn, New York, Pfaffmann pursued a distinguished academic career. He received an M.Sc. from Brown University in 1935 and, as a Rhodes scholar, went on to England's Oxford University. There, in 1937, he received a B.A. in animal physiology and biochemistry. He then took the marvelous opportunity of becoming a research student at Cambridge University, England under the famous Lord Adrian, one of the first and best electrophysiologists. From his distinguished tutor, Pfaffmann learned to refine his skill of placing electrodes into single sensory fibers and recording the nervous impulses produced when those receptors were stimulated.

Pfaffmann began his career as an electrophysiologist in search of the four receptor types that would correspond to the four

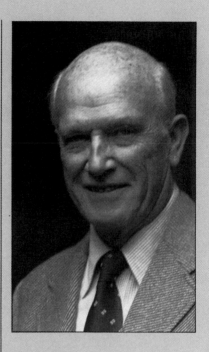

primary tastes — sweet, sour, salt and bitter — but soon found that no such correspondence existed. In 1941, however, he became one of the first scientists to record extensively the impulses along a single gustatory nerve fiber, after the taste receptor cells associated with it had been chemically stimulated.

In the years following, Pfaffmann and his colleagues pioneered the electro-physiology of taste. They painstakingly recorded the neural responses of taste receptors to various chemical stimuli, such as sugar, salt and hydrochloric acid, and found

that individual nerve fibers showed responses to two or more types of stimuli. Such findings posed questions about how taste receptors discriminate one taste stimulus from another. To explain this, Pfaffmann proposed a pattern, or ratio, theory. Simply stated, this suggests that the taste of a certain substance is coded in a pattern of different neural responses among a population of gustatory nerve fibers.

One of the most renowned physiological psychologists, Carl Pfaffmann has inspired a generation of workers in his field. Apart from his special interest in the sensory codes of neural impulses and the gustatory pathways to the brain, he has also experimented widely on many other aspects of taste.

Overall, Carl Pfaffmann's aim has been to mold a unified science of gustation, combining the three traditions of sensory electrophysiology, psycho-physics and psychobiology. His laboratory at Rockefeller University, New York, where he became Professor and academic Vice-President in 1965, has long been a beacon in the world of physiological psychology; a beacon kept blazing by his many students and fellow workers.

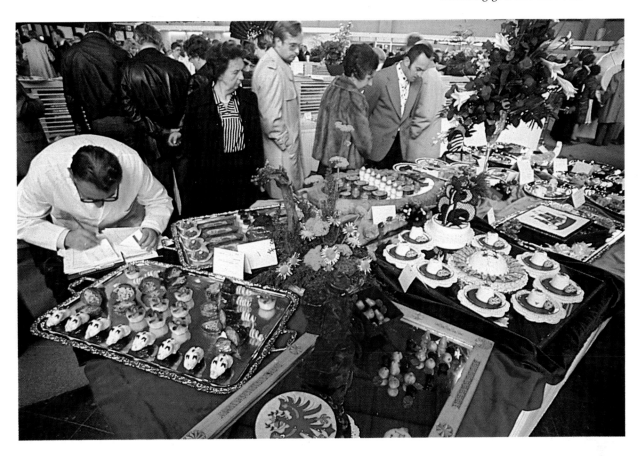

this day. There is little doubt that the taste buds do contain receptor cells that signal information about taste characteristics to the central nervous system. In the interweaving and interacting mix of receptor cells and nerve endings in each bud, however, it is still difficult to determine which of several possible candidates possesses the actual receptor surfaces where receptor potentials are generated.

What does a taste bud consist of? It is a cluster of perhaps thirty to eighty nonnervous cells, probably of ectodermal, epithelial origin, many of which have intimate connections with nerve endings. In humans, a cluster is about 20 to 40 microns wide and 60 to 70 microns high. As a micron is only one-thousandth of a millimeter, taste buds are clearly not things we are aware of bumping into while brushing our teeth. Indeed, the buds do not protrude above the general epithelial surface of the papillae at all, but are buried in the superficial cell layers and only communicate with the outside via

a narrow apical pore, usually 1 micron or less in diameter.

Much of the detailed knowledge about the cellular structure of taste buds in mammals has stemmed from the work of a relatively small, but select, group of research teams. Among these must be listed those under the direction of Lloyd M. Beidler at the Department of Biological Science, Florida State University; Carl Pfaffmann of the Rockefeller University, New York; and Raymond G. Murray of the Department of Anatomy and Physiology at Indiana University, Bloomington. The studies carried out by these groups on the ultrastructure, degeneration and regeneration of buds, with electron microscopical techniques (including e.m. cytochemistry) and with pulse labeling methodology, using isotopically labeled molecules, have in the past twenty years or so utterly transformed our knowledge of these tiny receptor units. Such work seems even more amazing when one considers that

The papillae-covered upper surface of the tongue is a world of astonishing three-dimensional complexity. A startling landscape of shapes is created by the various papillae: fringe-ended filiforms, rounded fungiforms and, most complex of all, the vallates. Taste buds are here visible as ovoid clusters of receptor cells, which are lodged in the epithelial walls of the fungiform and vallate papillae.

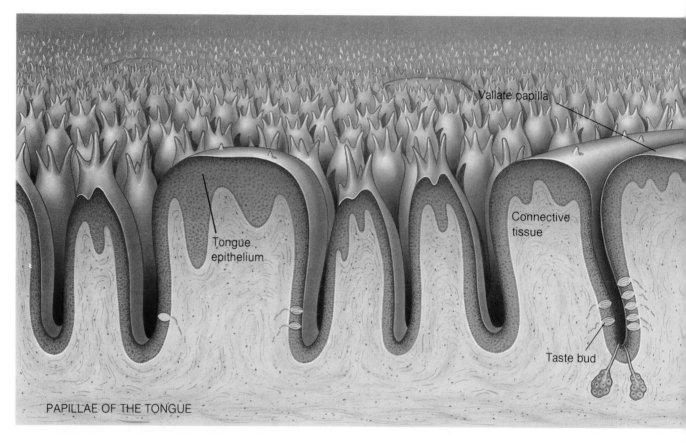

Vallate papilla

Tongue epithelium

Connective tissue

Taste bud

PAPILLAE OF THE TONGUE

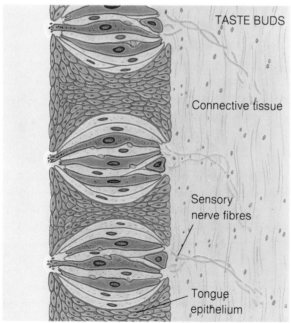

TASTE BUDS

Connective tissue

Sensory nerve fibres

Tongue epithelium

Each taste bud (left) is the interface between the sensory nerves that signal taste information to the brain, and the moist contents of the mouth cavity. Sweet, sour, salt and bitter substances in the mouth can only interact with receptor cells in the taste bud via an apical pore — a narrow channel between the bud cells and the contents of the mouth.

The detailed anatomy of a taste bud (right) reveals a cell pattern like the layers of an onion. The crucial components of the cell cluster are the three types of elongate cell, some of which are receptors and have close contacts with nerve endings.

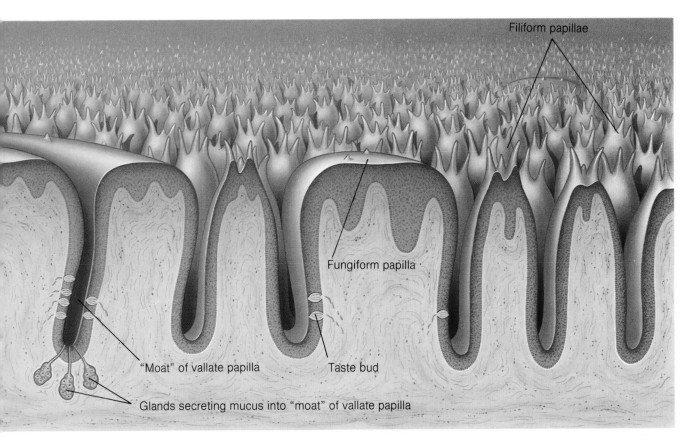

Filiform papillae

Fungiform papilla

"Moat" of vallate papilla

Taste bud

Glands secreting mucus into "moat" of vallate papilla

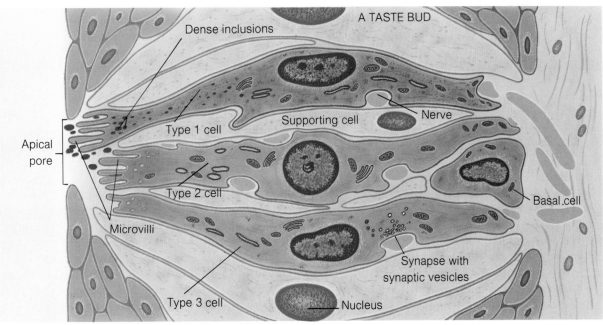

A TASTE BUD

Dense inclusions

Type 1 cell

Supporting cell

Nerve

Apical pore

Type 2 cell

Basal cell

Microvilli

Synapse with synaptic vesicles

Type 3 cell

Nucleus

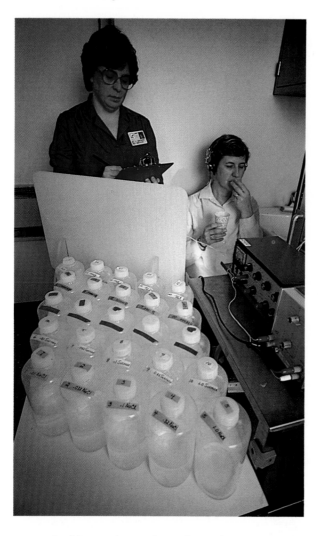

a taste bud is so minute that at least sixty or seventy could be packed together on one period from this page.

Minute as it is, the taste bud is seen through the electron microscope to be a sensory input device of high cellular complexity. In the body of the bud itself, there are three different cell types, which extend from the base of the bud upward to terminate in specialized microvillous endings (small finger-shaped projections) in the apical pore. These cells can be termed Types 1, 2 and 3 on the basis of their differing ultrastructural appearance. On first analysis, each of the cell types must be regarded as possible taste receptor cells because all three have extensive contacts with the fine nerve processes that penetrate the bud. All three, too, protrude into the external environment via the pore and could come into contact with taste stimuli. Differences in their structure, however, have lead some investigators to consider that other, nonsensory, functions may be carried out by at least one of the three types.

Inside a Taste Bud

Type 1 cells (also called dark cells), which constitute some 60 to 80 percent of the cell total, contain in their apical regions dark droplets, which seem to be extruded into the pore, providing a dense, mucoid coat around the microvillous tips of cell Types 1, 2 and 3. Type 1 cells have many contacts with nerve fibers, and some of these interactions bring nerves remarkably close to the nuclei of the cells. Moreover, they appear also to send processes around all the other cells of the bud. It is possible that these are not sensory cells at all but that they act instead as a supporting system for the other cells, in addition to elaborating the dense secretion within the pore.

Type 2 cells (15 to 30 percent of the cell total) and Type 3 cells (7 to 14 percent) have better structural credentials for being the real taste receptor cells. Type 2s, sometimes referred to as light cells, do not have secretory droplets but do possess particularly prominent sets of parallel microtubules and microfilaments, which extend from the microvilli at the cell tip deep into the cytoplasm. Type 3s have distinct synaptic contacts with nerve fibers but relatively simple tips — a synaptic contact is a junction between a nerve cell and another cell, across which signals can pass. As a working hypothesis, it seems reasonable to call Types 2 and 3 taste receptor cells and Type 1 a supporting cell. A fourth cell type within the bud, the basal cell, does not extend to the pore and is most unlikely to have a sensory function. It is conceivable that these basal cells are merely an early developmental stage of all the other cell types in a bud, but this theory is yet to be proved.

The development and dynamics of the cells of the bud are crucial to the understanding of the bud's function. Central to this understanding is the fact that the bud is in a state of flux, although it appears to be a structure with an unchanging composition. Just as a waterfall appears to be an entity but is composed of new water from moment to moment, so, too, is a taste bud composed of different cells from day to day. Isotopic pulse labeling experiments by Beidler have demonstrated conclusively that the cells of taste buds are constantly renewed; on average, they survive for only about ten days before being replaced. One interpretation of this renewal sequence is that cells around the edge of the bud divide by mitosis (the asexual division of one cell into two identical cells) to provide a source of new cells, which can enter the bud. Basal cells may well be newly arrived replacement cells, which then differentiate into Type 1, 2 and 3 cells. It is unlikely that Types 1, 2 and 3 can be converted from one to another because regeneration studies on denervated buds — ones whose nerve supply has been severed — show that as regeneration progresses, Types 1, 2 and 3 arise at approximately the same stage, suggesting that they do not develop sequentially.

Nerve Connections

In the embryological initiation of taste buds, their continuing existence and their regeneration, the role of the nerves is massive, indeed probably essential. The sensory nerve fibers of the relevant parts of the tongue, which have their cell bodies in the ganglia (aggregations of nerve cells) of the VIIth, IXth or Xth cranial nerves, are the crucial agents in this respect. As they grow into the surface layers of the developing tongue of a human fetus, they induce the production of taste bud cells and coordinate the organization of the buds.

As we have seen, taste receptor cells do not have their own nerve axon, but instead make extensive contacts with the ends of sensory nerve fibers. The continued existence of a bud through the whole of a human being's life depends on the presence of the nerve fiber array that brought it into being. If, for any reason of trauma or disease process, that connection between bud and nerves is broken, the bud rapidly degenerates. If, however, nerve axon regrowth into the epithelial layer is subsequently possible, the magical induction that occurred in embryonic life is reenacted in adulthood, and new taste buds form.

It is tempting to suggest that basal cells make contact with nerve fibers soon after they have

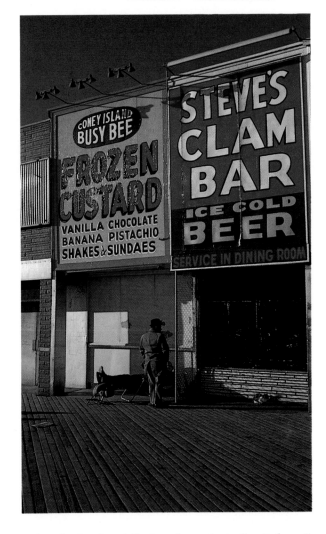

entered a bud and that such contacts "switch on" differentiation into cell Types 1, 2 and 3. But experiments have shown, first, that it is only the nerves (VII, IX and X) that normally innervate the taste buds which can bring about this induction, and, second, that epithelium from the lining of the front of the alimentary tract is necessary for the process to occur.

Having seen how taste buds populate the surface of the papillate region of the tongue and having considered the bewildering microcosm constituted by their cellular architecture, let us now look at their functional context. What do taste buds taste? How do they taste? And what role does the sense of taste play in our lives?

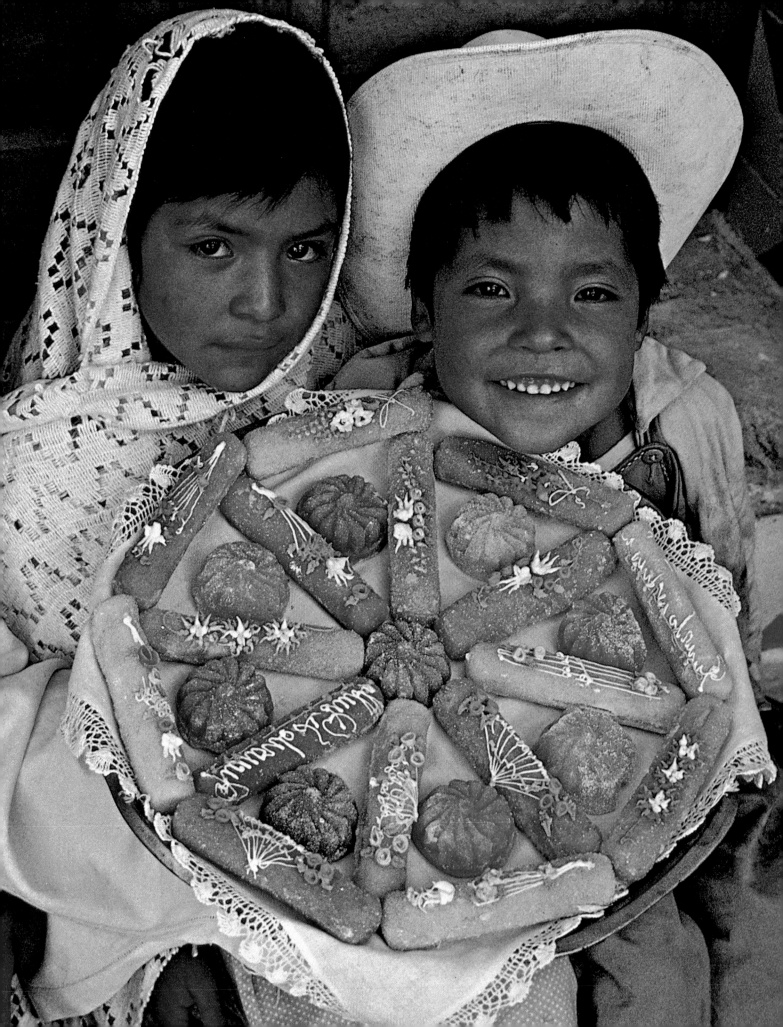

Chapter 5

Sweet, Sour, Salt, Bitter

What are little girls made of, made of?
What are little girls made of?
Sugar and spice
And all things nice,
That's what little girls are made of.

When the anonymous writer of the traditional nursery rhyme wanted to be complimentary about the nature of young ladies, nothing was more natural than to imagine that they were composed of sweet, tasty foods. Taste imagery pervades human consciousness; taste metaphors and taste analogies are constantly reiterated in any conversation about mood, personality, emotions, pleasurable or unhappy experiences.

People we like are said to be sweet, those we do not, sour. Orators and advertisers speak in honeyed tones. Someone who harbors a grudge is considered bitter. To be tasteful is the most refined of attributes, while something that is disapproved of is termed unwholesome. We perform with great gusto or show disgust — both words derive, like gustation itself, from the Latin for taste, *gustatus*.

It seems that the perceptions that we call taste are so powerful, so extensive in their capacity to conjure up clusters of associated feelings, that we freely transfer the language of taste to all other parts of our experience. But how does taste perception actually arise in the taste buds, sensory nerves and the brain? What are the limits of discrimination and sensitivity of this basic sense and its uses in human life and society?

The Qualities of Taste

The sense of taste evolved in relation to the response to food and has its greatest significance in this context. The sense with which we now tell the difference between real and artificial cream or between two varieties of wine was originally of value to our ancestors in choosing between, and recognizing, different natural food items —

Love of sweet-tasting substances is not confined to humans. All kinds of organisms, from bacteria and insects to most mammals, display a preference for sweetness. Although we often try to reverse this preference for the sake of our waistlines, the reason for its evolutionary development is clearly connected with the fact that naturally sweet substances tend to be important sources of calories, and they are, therefore, valuable, energy-providing foods.

85

Unripe fruit is usually sour and unpalatable. During the ripening process, starches break down into sugars, which mask acidity and create the sweet flavor so loved by man and other animals.

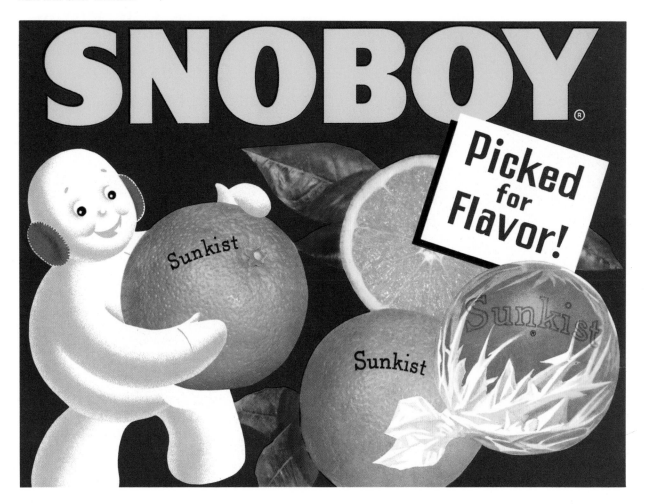

leaves, fruits, nuts, berries, tubers, roots, fungi and so on. Such choices could have been a matter of life and death. With appropriate past experience, a minute nibble from one of a cluster of mushrooms could have told one of our hunter-gatherer forerunners that the fungi were edible or extremely poisonous. Small wonder, under this type of selection pressure, that the sense of taste of such an omnivorous, opportunistic primate as man should have become so refined and subtle.

The sensory response to different types of molecule, centered on the taste buds of the tongue, is a vital part of total taste perception. But this chemoreception is not, by any means, the whole of our taste experience. Taste itself is associated with a range of other food qualities, which are perceived before and during the period that food is being consumed. The physical texture of the food, its resistance to chewing, the sound of it being chewed, its temperature and its smell, all fuse with taste into a complete sensory experience, referred to simply as taste.

Experience teaches us that taste chemoreception, by the taste buds of the tongue and other regions at the beginning of the alimentary tract, divides into broadly differing types of sensation. Although these tastes cannot be unambiguously defined in the same way that the wavelength of a particular colored light or the frequency of a sound can be specified, it is agreed that taste perception can be regarded as a chord of the chemical senses playable on four notes.

The notes are sweet, salt, sour (or acid) and bitter. It is likely that all tastes are generated by a

Direct tasting experiments have shown that different regions of the tongue have characteristically different levels of sensitivity to the four basic taste sensations: sweet, sour, salt and bitter.

THE FOUR TASTE SENSATIONS

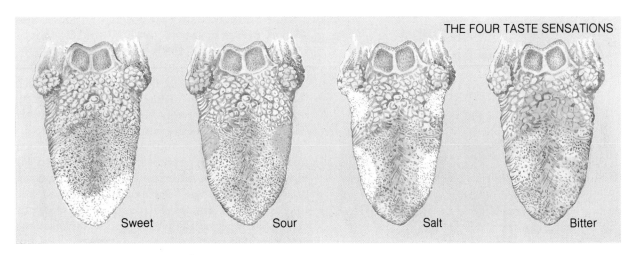

Sweet   Sour   Salt   Bitter

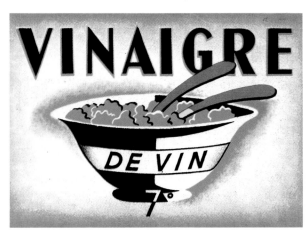

The sour taste of vinegar makes a sharp counterpart to bland oily substances and improves their flavor, hence its use in sauces and salad dressings. The main acidic component in vinegar is acetic acid — an oxidation component of alcohol, which is itself made by the fermentation of any sugar by yeasts or bacteria. Malt vinegars are made in this way from the sugars in malted barley; wine vinegars from grape sugars and alcohol. Wine vinegars are generally considered to have the best flavor.

combination of these four notes in differing intensities. It is important, however, to remember that the substances themselves — sugar, sea salt, orange juice, tonic water — are not flavored. Taste is not a quality of materials but a modeling of some features of the chemical composition of those substances within the human nervous system. That modeling is perceived as taste and localized to the areas where the taste buds and materials come into contact.

The different types of papillae on the tongue show some area-specific patterns of taste selectivity. Essentially, fungiform papillae respond only to sweet and salt tastes, while the vallate papillae at the back of the papilla-covered region of the tongue are much more sensitive to sour and bitter food qualities. The foliate receptors at the sides of the tongue are also tuned to respond predominantly to sourness. Thus, a characteristic contour map of the surface of the tongue shows that the sides have peak sensitivity to acidic tastes, the free tip to sugars, while the back of the papillate zone of the tongue is most sensitive to bitterness. The common experience that some sweetish substances, such as saccharin, have a bitter aftertaste is partly a result of the journey of that substance from the front to back of the tongue. The sweet taste is experienced first because of the tip's sensitivity, but this sweetness is then mixed with a bitter taste as the vallate papillae positioned at the back of the tongue respond to the stimulus.

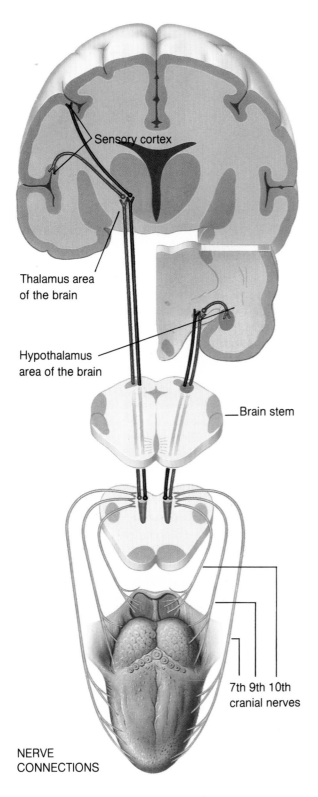

Sensory cortex

Thalamus area
of the brain

Hypothalamus
area of the brain

Brain stem

7th 9th 10th
cranial nerves

NERVE
CONNECTIONS

Taste buds on the tongue itself are supplied with sensory nerves by cranial nerves VII and IX. Cranial nerve VII, also called the facial nerve, provides the innervation for the front regions of the tongue in front of the transverse groove. The neural branch that carries out this role is the chorda tympani, referred to in the previous chapter, and it is mainly concerned with nerve impulses signaling information about salt and sweet taste sensations from the fungiform papillae in the front two-thirds of the tongue. The IXth cranial nerve, the glosso-pharyngeal, supplies the posterior part of the tongue and is the route along which nervous activity corresponding to bitter and sour sensations is transmitted from the taste buds of the vallate and foliate papillae. The scattered taste buds distributed on the palate, epiglottis, uvula, larynx and upper portions of the esophagus gain their sensory nerve supply from the Xth cranial nerve, the vagus.

How Taste Buds Work
The generally accepted framework for understanding the manner in which the receptor cells in taste buds do their job relies on the central idea that the stimulus chemicals in the mouth (tastant molecules) interact with the cell membranes of the projections of receptor cells in the apical pore of taste buds. By attachment to the cell surface, or perhaps by other types of contact, the tastant molecules are presumed to induce short-term changes in the

The rich interlinkings of nerves between the tongue and the central nervous system are extraordinarily complex. This composite image shows in a stylized form the way in which sensory nerve fibers in cranial nerves VII, IX and X course back into the brain stem. The pathways of nerves to higher levels of the brain are also stylized for clarity. Links are made on both sides of the real brain with the subcortical regions (shown only on the right of the diagram) and the cerebral cortex (shown only on the left).

All the molecules illustrated taste sweet to human tongues, despite the range of organic molecule categories to which they belong. It is thought that they share an ability to elicit a sweet taste because, in their molecular structure, they all contain one or more so-called AH,B atomic groupings. These are thought to interact with special proteins in the receptor cell membranes to elicit a sweet taste response.

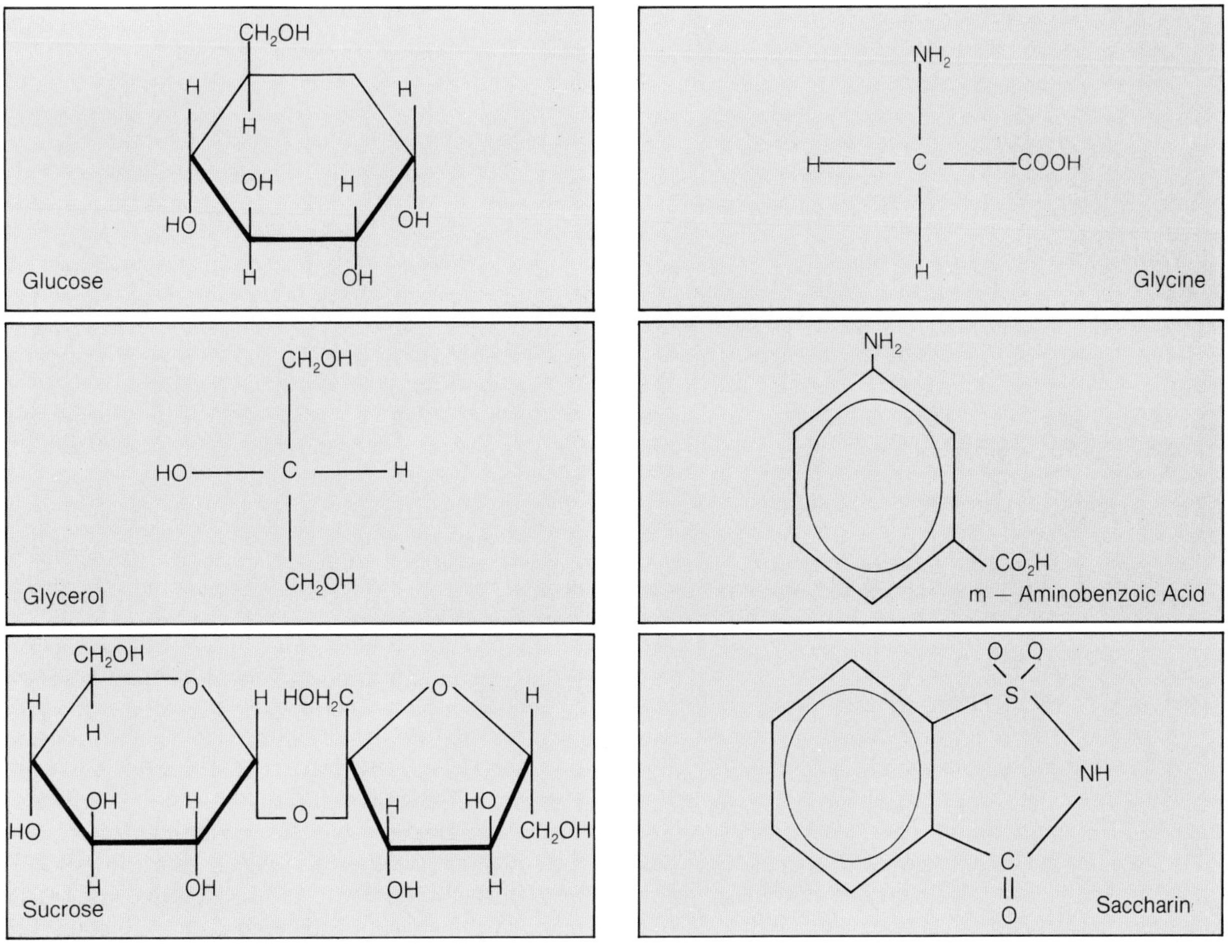

Glucose

Glycine

Glycerol

m — Aminobenzoic Acid

Sucrose

Saccharin

permeability of the receptor cell membrane. Such changes bring about movements across the membrane of charged ions, which generate electrical disturbances. These in turn induce the initiation of trains of nerve impulses in the sensory nerve endings closely associated with the receptor cells in the taste bud. By such a series of linked causes and effects, the presence of a particular tastant molecule in the apical pore — the aperture by which taste buds communicate with the external environment — is matched with corresponding sensory nerve impulses.

A great deal of experimental work, using human subjects but more often other mammals such as rats or cats, has been carried out on the above theory, to try and unravel the practical physiological and molecular details of these basic receptor processes.

One important strand of this work has concentrated on a search for those receptor molecules in the cell membrane of receptor cells which could be involved in "lock and key" couplings with particular types of tastant molecules. The nodal ideal behind the philosophy of such work is that a particular chemical or electronic grouping, shared by a range of different chemicals, could link up selectively with a receptor molecule in the receptor membrane; this could mean that all such chemicals would share a particular taste. Investigations have been particularly successful in respect of the perception of sweet tastes, many of the more substantial advances in this area stemming from the researches of Dr. R. S. Shallenberger and his associates from the Agricultural Research Service at Beltsville, Maryland.

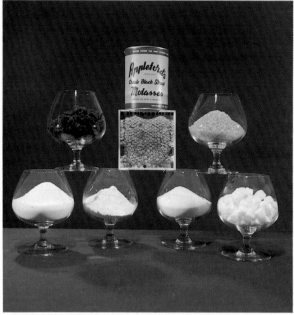

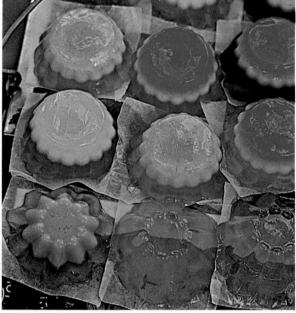

A crucial year in the development of these ideas was 1967, when Dr. Shallenberger and his colleague Dr. T. E. Acree published their general theory for the chemical characteristic that was common to all sweet-tasting substances. Rejoicing in the name of the AH,B theory of taste, it proposed that all molecules that elicit a sweet taste response via taste buds possess an electronegative atom (A), often oxygen or nitrogen, with that atom being linked by a single bond to a positive hydrogen nucleus or proton. The −OH (hydroxyl) groups, with which all ordinary sugars are richly endowed, constitute such AH entities. For the grouping to be able to elicit a sweet taste, the theory suggested that, very close to the proton, there must exist another electronegative atom (B), again, normally an oxygen or nitrogen atom. The gap between the proton and B is crucial; it must be extremely narrow, less, in fact, than 3 Ångstrom units, that is less than ·0000003 millimeters or three ten-millionths of a millimeter.

The theory assumes that the AH,B grouping is necessary for the locking together of the sweet tastant molecules and a receptor molecule for such tastants in the receptor membrane. It explains also the sweetness elicited by substances such as sugars, saccharin, cyclamate, amino acids, lead acetate and some salts of beryllium — they all possess the crucial AH,B pattern.

More recently, firm evidence has been forthcoming that a protein, bound to the surface-membrane, is the sweet-tastant receptor molecule. A protein-containing fraction has been extracted from the epithelial layers of cows' tongues that can specifically form complexes with substances known to elicit a sweet sensation. Even before the isolation of such good protein candidates for the role of sweet-tastant receptor molecules, indirect evidence existed that all sweet stimuli act by way of a common receptor mechanism.

The Taste Changers

Gymnemic acid, a complex organic compound, can be extracted from the leaves of an Indian plant, *Gymnema sylvestre*. When taken by mouth, gymnemic acid has the remarkable property of temporarily suppressing the sensitivity of taste buds to sweet stimuli. Dr. Kenso Kurihara, from the Faculty of Science of the Tokyo Institute of Technology, has made an intensive study of taste modifiers like gymnemic acid. He gives a succinct description of the effect of chewing the leaves: "If one chews the leaves... sugar tastes much like sand and sugar solution tastes like tap water." What is particularly

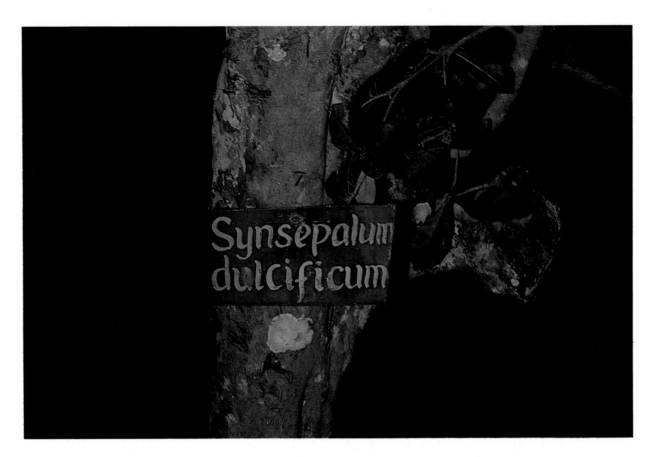

fascinating is that Dr. Kurihara has shown that the ability of this substance to suppress the perception of sweetness extends to the vast majority of chemical types of sweet tastants. For gymnemic acid abolishes the sweetness of beryllium chloride, lead acetate, D-amino acids and cyclamate just as well as it does that of sucrose or glucose.

Yet another astounding taste modifier is the miracle fruit, *Synsepalum dulcificum,* a plant that grows in West Africa and produces olive-sized red berries. These berries are aptly named miracle fruit, and the specific name of the plant, *dulcificum,* "sweetening," signals the nature of the miracle. For centuries, the inhabitants of West African countries, such as Ghana, have chewed the berries for their effect of converting sour tastes to sweet. If miracle fruits are chewed before taking traditional foods such as sour maize bread or acidic palm wine, both taste sweet. Even a lemon can be munched like a sweet orange.

Kurihara and the American scientist Beidler have extracted the active ingredient of the berries and found it to be a glycoprotein, that is, a protein with sugar molecules bound to it. The glycoprotein of the miracle fruit contains almost 7 percent of sugar components, identified as the monosaccharides arabinose and xylose. How can this substance in-

duce up to three hours worth of sour to sweet taste conversion when swilled round the mouth at extremely low concentrations?

The following interpretation not only explains the phenomenon but also fits in with the theory of receptor sites for sweet-tastant molecules detailed above. It is assumed that the miracle fruit protein can attach itself to the surface of a taste receptor cell close to the site of a sweet receptor protein. The presence of a sour stimulus will always entail an increase in acidity. It then seems likely that this increase induces a shape change in the miracle fruit protein, causing one or other of its attached sugar molecules (arabinose or xylose) to move and interact with the receptor site on the sweet receptor protein. This induces a sweet sensation, lasting as long as the acidic substances are present.

Salt, Sour and Bitter Tastes
Clearly, there is now a considerable amount known about the sensory transduction (conversion of stimuli into nervous events) that occurs with respect to sweet-tastant molecules. To what extent can this knowledge be extrapolated to the other three taste types: salt, sour and bitter? For salt tastes, there are two somewhat different theories in existence at present.

Lloyd Beidler

Demystifying Taste

One of the world's foremost experts on taste, Lloyd Beidler, with the help of twentieth-century technology such as the electron microscope, has looked far more closely at the interface between chemicals and the tongue than any other scientist before him.

Born in 1922, in Allentown, Pennsylvania, Beidler began his academic career as a physicist, spending from 1944 to 1946 working at the Radiation Laboratory, Johns Hopkins University. In 1950, he joined the Florida State University, Tallahassee, where he is now Professor of Physiology.

Beidler's fascination with taste has been focused mainly on the interaction of molecules: what is there in sweet, sour, salty or bitter substances that triggers off such individual taste sensations? And what can be found out about receptor cells and their membranes that will lead to a better understanding of how taste works? There is still much more to discover, as Beidler would be the first to admit, but his research has placed knowledge about gustation on a firm, twentieth-century footing.

In 1956, Beidler and his colleagues reported that, just as a population of nerve fibers

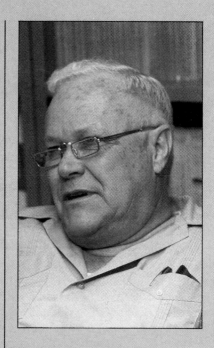

leaving the taste buds shows multiple sensitivity (a fact which Carl Pfaffmann and others had shown previously), so do the individual receptor cells in the taste bud. In other words, one and the same chemoreceptor cell will react to different substances, such as salt and sucrose, or salt and hydrochloric acid. As a result of experiments, Beidler realized that taste receptor cells are not rigidly specific, as was once believed, but are sensitive to all substances in varying degrees.

In the early 1960s Beidler continued to try and demystify the sense of taste: by using a process of radioactively labeling the DNA of the cells in and around a taste bud, he showed that taste bud cells are constantly being renewed. He found that cells around the edge of the bud divide by mitosis and appear to provide a source of new cells. Having entered the bud, new cells migrate toward the center as they age and are briefly active as receptor cells before disintegrating.

Yet another important area of Lloyd Beidler's work has concerned the transduction of salty tastes — he discovered that a salty taste arises when the cation, or positive part of the salt, temporarily alters the structure of a receptor membrane protein and triggers an electrical response along the sensory nerve fiber. He also investigated the way in which sweetness and sourness are transferred from stimulus to perception. His work on these topics has demonstrated that different animal species have different electrophysiological responses to various taste stimuli.

In these and many other research projects, Beidler has been one of the greatest contributors to twentieth-century knowledge of taste and has vastly improved our understanding of this hitherto neglected sense.

The first theory, largely associated with Lloyd M. Beidler of Florida State University, is compatible with the sweet stimulus system already described. Like that, it assumes that receptor proteins in the cell membrane of taste receptor cells interact with salt stimuli. Salt-tasting substances are, in the main, molecules that in water break up into separate positively and negatively charged ionic fragments: cations and anions respectively. Experiments with salts containing the same cation, but different anions, at equal ionic concentrations, have led Beidler to conclude that it is cations like that of sodium ($Na+$) that stimulate the receptor proteins responsible for salt tastes, whereas the negatively charged anions are probably inhibitory. In the same way as in the sweet transduction story, it is assumed that ion concentrations induce shape changes in the receptor proteins, which ultimately bring about sensory nerve impulses.

The second theory on the mechanism of salt taste turns to nonprotein constituents of the receptor cell membranes as a target for the salt stimuli. At a molecular level, membranes are composed of a double layer of part-charged, part-fatty molecules called phospholipids. This bilayer provides the framework of the membrane in which are embedded a variety of proteins and glycoproteins. The idea of this second theory is that the cationic salt stimuli become associated with the charged parts of the phospholipid layer in the first phases of the transduction of salty tastes.

Sour stimulus transduction, the first events that occur on the tongue when we taste lemon juice or a vinegary salad dressing or bite into a tart apple, again appear to be linked to receptor proteins. In this instance, it is positively charged hydrogen ions ($H+$) from acids that can induce shape changes in the protein. It is interesting here to note that it is exactly this form of acidity-induced alteration in protein shape that is thought to account for the amazing properties of the miracle fruit.

Bitter-tasting substances, like sweet ones, come in a wide spectrum of chemical families. Unlike the sweet stimuli, however, it has so far been impossible to recognize any single atomic or electronic set of ground rules for predicting with some accuracy which molecules will be bitter and which will not. Natural protective organic molecules synthesized

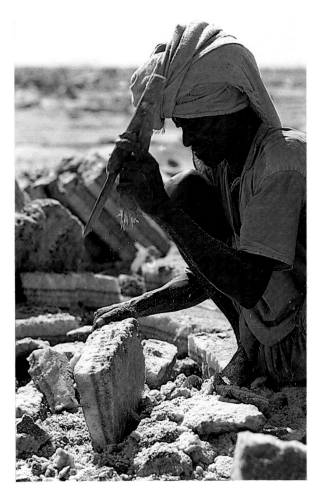

by plants (sometimes termed secondary compounds) are often bitter tasting. In this category are alkaloids, such as quinine, caffeine, cocaine, strychnine and nicotine, as well as diterpenes and some glycosides.

Consider now, the fascinating sensory and evolutionary "dialogue" which has been going on between plant-eating animals and the plants themselves for so many million years. It is likely that the sweet-bitter divergence in our taste capabilities is the result of this plant-animal interaction. Sugars of all types are the classic, energy-rich substances produced by plants and, as such, are an efficient resource for feeding animals to use. What more reasonable evolutionary direction than for animals to produce a generalized taste sensation that equates with the presence of the multiple $-OH$

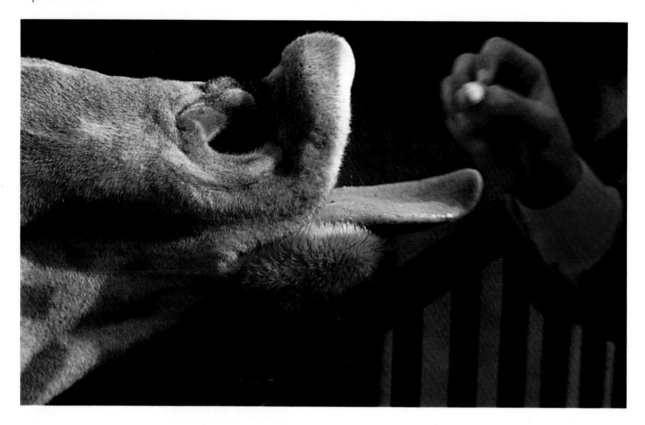

groups on sugars — that is, the sweet taste? Furthermore, in an extraordinarily wide range of organisms from single-celled types up to man himself, sweet stimuli are attractive and almost always induce feeding activity.

What of the other side of the bitter-sweet coin? The bitter-tasting secondary compounds constructed by plants discourage potential consumers. Herbivores, from minute moth caterpillars to giraffes, may be dissuaded from eating leaves containing such substances. As so many of the compounds are definitely toxic — think of deadly nightshade or poison ivy — it is obviously advantageous for animals to have a sensitive and generalized capacity with regard to these hazardous "natural food additives." Many sensory biologists believe that the bitter taste faculty is exactly such a capacity. For almost all animals, man included, bitter is a taste to be avoided and spit out.

There is no real scientific consensus about bitterness transduction, although it seems plausible that bitter tastants first interact with the membrane phospholipids. However, genetical findings relating to "taste blindness" suggest that there is some crucial protein involvement, either direct or indirect. A varying proportion of human populations find an organic molecule called PTC (phenylthiocarbamide) either intensely bitter or almost completely tasteless.

The sensitivity to this type of bitterness is controlled by a single Mendelian dominant gene. "Taste blind" individuals have the double recessive gene mix (tt), while those with double dominant (TT) or dominant/recessive (Tt) mixes find PTC bitter. The simplest explanation of such findings assumes that the T gene is coding for a functional receptor protein for this type of bitterness. Those "taste blind" to PTC are fully sensitive to all other taste types, including (and this is a crucial piece of evidence) other molecular types of bitterness. Thus, from this research, it would seem that the human tongue receptor cells bear a number of different bitter sensitivities, although all are perceived as the same "bitter" taste sensation.

A vital organ, the muscular tongue moves food around the mouth during chewing and shapes it into a mass for swallowing. Without it, not only could we not lick an ice cream, we could not eat solid food at all.

The trains of nerve impulses that flood back along the sensory nerves from the taste buds to the brain are not yet taste sensation. The latter is a perception generated by the conscious portions of the mind. How, though, do the nerve signals from the tongue undergo central nervous system processing in order to produce localized taste sensations — a sweet taste at the tip of the tongue, for example? And how is the taste information utilized to coordinate and control particular patterns of behavior such as eating?

At present there are only the outlines of answers to these fundamental questions. Despite the imprecision of our understanding, the evidence that does exist reveals a vivid impression of the miraculously intricate interconnections of our nervous system. It also illustrates the manner in which this supremely efficient microcircuitry handles the input of sensory data.

Taking nervous processes in a taste-bud-to-brain sequence, it is the clusters of sensory nerve impulses that must be scrutinized first. Contrary to what might be imagined about the individual sensory nerve fibers, they do not each carry information about a single taste type — salt, sour, sweet or bitter — alone. When one records electrophysiologically from single fibers in, for example, the chorda tympani nerve, while stimulating the tongue with different tastant molecules, it is rapidly obvious that a single chorda tympani axon is not specifically sensitive to a particular taste stimulus type. What is found is that each fiber has a characteristic quantitive capacity to respond to almost all taste types. It is as though each fiber has a particular signature of sensitivities to different tastes.

If this last statement is true, as it seems to be, the central processing of sensory taste impulses must be on the level of populations of fibers rather than individual ones. The central nervous system appears to survey the overall pattern of incoming sensory impulses and to take a "weighted average" of their taste messages as the perceived taste. The weighting must, in such an instance, depend on the pattern of firing among a population of fibers, some of which are most responsive to salt, others to sugar and so on. These fibers have graded, rather than all-or-nothing, sensitivities to the four taste types.

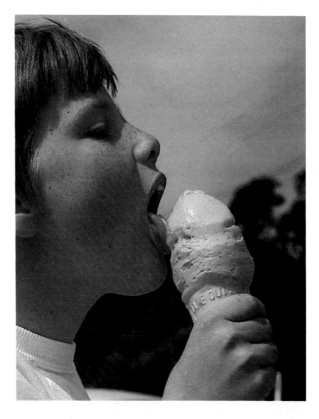

The psychophysiology of taste tends to confirm this concept of nerve impulse processing at a conscious level. When we experience a complex, multi-component flavor, we usually report a unified, complete-in-itself taste. If asked to describe the characteristics of the total taste, subjects do not say that it is half salt, a quarter sweet and a quarter bitter. The answer might be something like, "It tastes like slightly moldy oranges." In other words, a single taste that can only be described verbally in terms of other complex tastes. As if to support this perceptual evidence, attempts to find individual fibers that respond to only one taste type in the consciousness-related cortical parts of the brain have all failed.

The complex routes, technically the central gustatory projections, by which taste sensory inputs enter the central nervous system can be divided into two main tracks. First, there are the so-called subcortical connections, which route incoming signals from the receptors to evolutionarily ancient brain stem regions such as the medulla and

A critical chef samples a sauce, probably unconsciously taking account of its smell and texture as well as its taste, in order to make a subtle judgment as to the correct balance of flavors.

In J. F. de Troy's painting Oyster Feast, *diners gorge themselves on the delicious shellfish. Oysters have a distinct tinge of the sea in their flavor, which is refreshing and stimulating to the palate.*

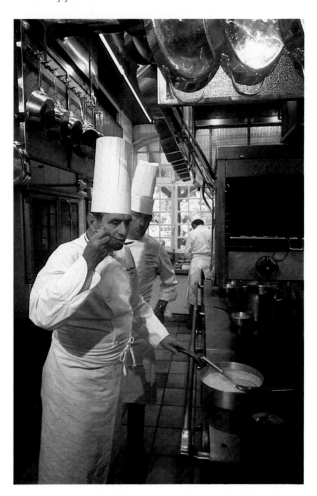

cerebellum. Using a variety of investigative methods including microelectrode recording and the tracing of injected radioisotopes, it has been shown that the subcortical projections involve nerve cells located in the solitary tract of the medulla, within the region of the brain called the pons, and within the general area of the amygdala and lateral hypothalamus. The functional significance of these types of connection is to be sought in nonconscious, stereotyped links between some types of taste information and behavior.

Instinctive Responses

We are aware of the power of these instinctual imperatives in animals such as rats. In experiments, even a decerebrate rat (one that has had its cerebrum removed and is thus incapable of using

its higher brain functions) is still perfectly capable of an instinctive response when sugar solution is placed on its tongue. Without any conscious control, this stimulus elicits feeding behavior. In the terrible congenital abnormality of human babies termed anencephaly, the cerebral cortex does not develop; yet in these decerebrate children some basic, instinctive responses to tastes remain. Human beings are apparently programed at a nonconscious level to respond positively to sweet stimuli and to reject bitter ones, despite the fact that we may consciously reprogram ourselves to reverse these preferences.

The fact that nonconscious taste inputs route to the amygdala and hypothalamus areas of the brain is particularly significant because other brain function experiments have told us much about these zones, buried low in the cranium. In animals that chase and kill other animals for food, as man himself has always done, parts of the amygdala are intimately concerned with the control of the killing of prey. Other portions of the amygdala are linked to the nonconscious control of gut functions such as intestinal peristalsis and the secretion of gastric acid and digestive enzymes.

Similarly, the lateral hypothalamus seems to exert some overall control on feeding behavior and appetite. Interest in foodstuffs, levels of food consumption and the maintenance of a particular body weight are all processes with which the hypothalamus has been linked. Given this interrelated pattern of functions linked to food and feeding in these parts of the brain, it is especially appropriate that sensory data on tastes in the mouth should be routed there. It is conceivable, too, that some of the information directed thus should come from taste sensory nerves that are unusually specific in their responses to one of the four taste qualities.

If this last hypothesis is true, it is possible that we and other higher vertebrates respond to tastes in two rather disparate ways. There may well be a few nerve "hot lines," rapidly conducting pathways that carry simple signals — salt, sour, sweet, bitter — to the nonconscious lower brain, which is the control center for our instinctive taste responses. Such rapid, unconscious internal signaling would, for instance, switch on a baby's sucking

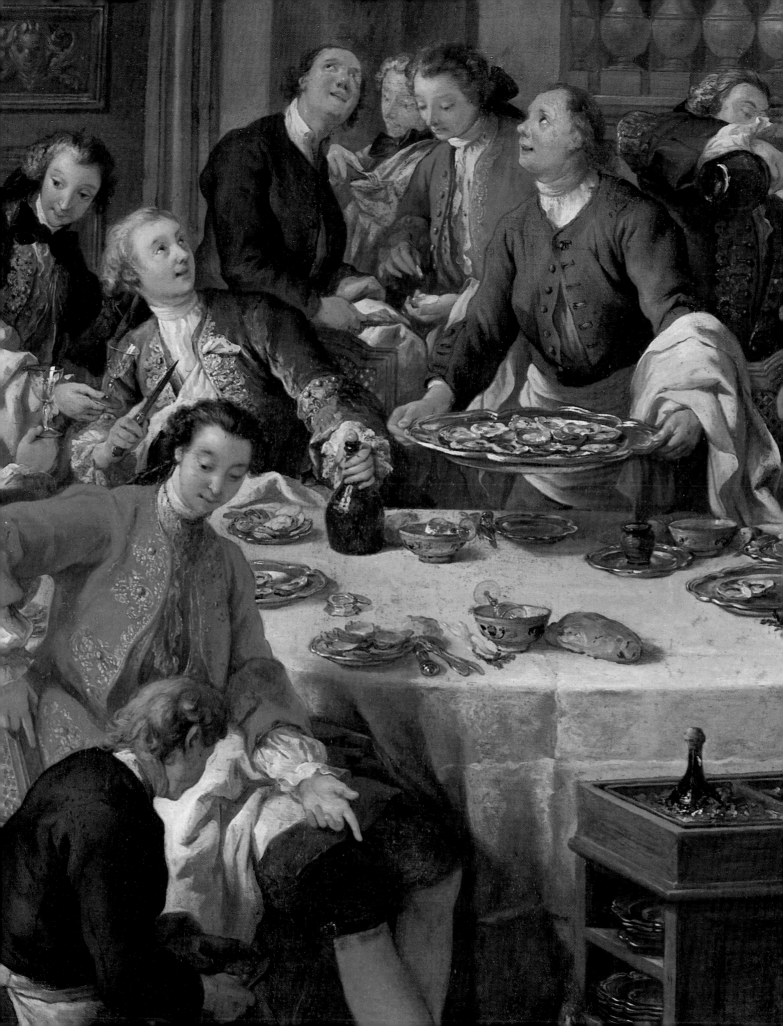

*A lavish feast of fruits, suckling pig
and other delicacies spread in a
tropical setting, appeals to the eye as
well as to the taste buds. Flavorsome
food should always be aesthetically
pleasing.*

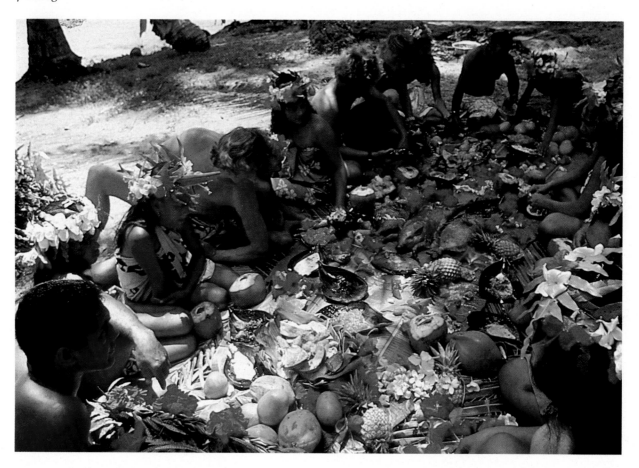

reflex when warm, sweet breast milk is in its mouth or make it reject sour milk in a bottle.

In contrast, the patterns of activity in the nerves that can carry information about all types of taste stimulus are extremely complex. These nerve activity patterns do reach the conscious levels of our minds and are responsible for the direct perception that we have of taste. They are also involved with all our fine discriminations between one taste and another, as well as with consciously motivated changes in our instinctive responses to taste. Think of the mesh of feelings, social pressures, self-image, appetite and a dozen other factors which may make a person desire, but consciously reject, sweet foods while on a calorie-controlled diet, and the full complexity of conscious taste response reprograming becomes obvious.

Just as the subcortical projections of taste have been well charted by neurophysiologists and

neurologists, so too have the turnpikes of nerves that take taste information to our brain's cerebral cortex, the so-called cortical projections. The fibers identified in this way pass into a taste "nucleus" in the basal regions of the thalamus and from there outward radiating to at least two separate regions of the cortex. Links within the cortex integrate taste information with other types of sensory input. In particular, the separate senses of taste and touch on the tongue will be coordinated at these higher brain levels, and the location of a taste in the mouth is perceived there.

Taste Appraisal
Perhaps the easiest way of explaining the full richness of the links between taste and human behavior, of exemplifying the massive sensitivity and subtlety of human gustatory abilities, is to look at a single complex task — that of the professional

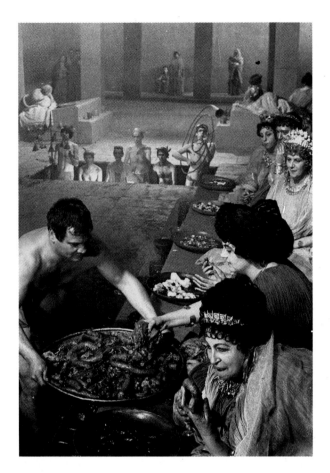

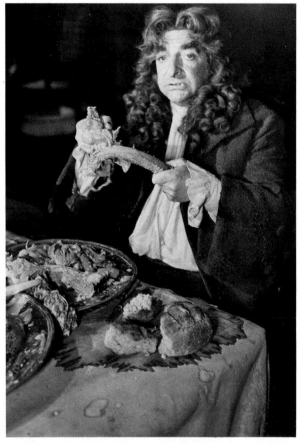

wine taster. Such a person is capable of specifically identifying a wine to the extent of the grape variety, year, location of the vineyard and, maybe, even the producer, simply by having a glass in his or her hand and then tasting a mouthful. Appearance, smell (bouquet) and taste (palate) combine with years of experience to achieve this marvel of sensory integration. As T.G. Shaw wrote 120 years ago in a book entitled *Wine, the Vine and the Cellar*, "...the palate, like the eye, the ear, or touch, acquires with practice various degrees of sensitiveness that would be incredible were it not a well ascertained fact."

Taste is the last of three phases in a wine taster's appreciation. Only after the appearance of the wine has been examined for its color, depth and clarity, and its bouquet savored and defined, will a mouthful be tasted. Professionals know all about the different areas of taste sensitivity on the tongue.

Michael Broadbent, an eminent writer on the subject of wine, writes "... to take a very small sip or leave only the tip of the tongue in contact, will not enable the taster to appreciate more than a fraction of the wine's physical characteristics. A reasonable mouthful must be taken and it must be swirled round the mouth so that all the taste buds can get to work on it."

The vocabulary of the wine taster, like that of any specialized professional, appears to the outsider to be jargon-stuffed and complicated. Such complexity has evolved in response to the need to describe a range of finely demarcated attributes which non-experts simply do not recognize. Again from the pen of Michael Broadbent, the palate section of a description of a "blind-tasted" 1966 Châteauneuf-du-Pape: "Very slight sweetness for a red (i.e. not austerely dry like many a Medoc). As full-bodied as it looks: heavy in the mouth, revealing considerable

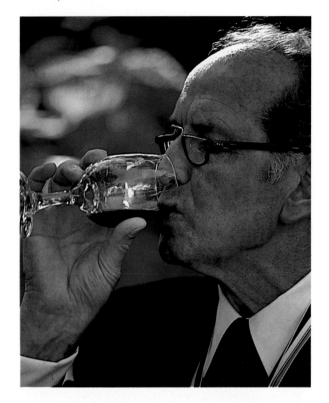

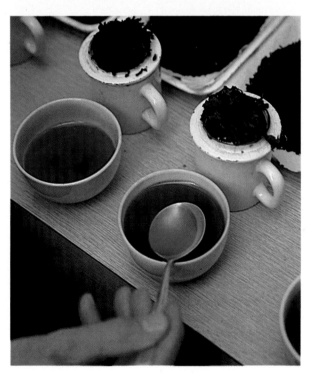

weight of alcohol, and full of extract. Robust yet curiously soft (lacking the excess tannin and acidity of a Bordeaux of the same weight and youthfulness). A nice, slightly scented flavor; still a little raw, and with a faintly bitter finish.''

The language of wine has often been mocked and found pretentious. Yet this description, with its linked data on color and bouquet, enabled the taster precisely to identify this wine. Who could mock in the face of such accomplishment?

Little is known of the detailed way in which a wine taster is able to make minutely specific discriminations between closely related wines by pure sensory deduction. Experiment can, however tell us something of the absolute sensitivities to differing taste qualities. The minimum threshold concentrations at which substances can just be distinguished from water alone have been determined on a number of occasions. These thresholds are usually expressed as molarities, where a molarity of 1 represents the molecular weight in grams of the substance dissolved in a liter of water. Expressed in this way, some sensitivity thresholds are remarkably low. The most sensitive individuals can perceive hydrochloric acid (an acid taste) at 0.00005 M and sodium chloride (salt taste) at 0.001 M. Similarly, a range of sweet substances is first noticed at the following concentration levels: sucrose, 0.005 M; glucose, 0.04 M and saccharin 0.00002 M; while some people can still taste quinine sulphate (the substance that makes tonic water bitter) at a level of 0.0000004 M.

Altered Perceptions

One facet of the complexity of human taste perception is the way in which taste sensitivity and judgments about the acceptability of certain flavors are altered by both our physiological state and our health. As we have seen, taste does give us direct information about some aspects of the nutritional quality of foods. Partly as a result of this channel of information flow, infants are able to choose a balanced and sustaining diet with no direct adult intervention. So-called ''cafeteria'' experiments, in which children were allowed to make their own food choices from a wide range of natural foodstuffs, have demonstrated this point conclusively.

Tests also prove that sodium-depleted persons

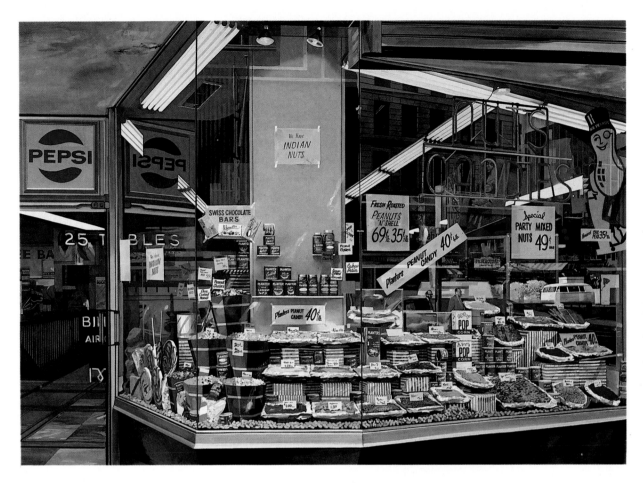

(and animals) show a specific hunger for salty food. To people who are not short of salt, low salt concentrations taste pleasant and acceptable, while higher levels are unpalatable and, indeed, are likely to be toxic. In a salt-depleted person, the threshold of salt acceptability climbs so that very salty foods are thought to be attractively flavored despite the fact that they would normally be inedible.

Taste perception can also be altered during many diseases, and there are at least two mechanisms for such changes. The first is little to do with taste *per se*. In a wide range of respiratory infections, increased nasal secretion of mucus greatly reduces the efficiency of the sense of smell but also affects taste, making food seem dull and insipid. Much of this change is probably caused by the removal of the smell component from our sense of "taste."

The second mechanism for changing taste perception in illness is concerned with taste itself. It is the phenomenon of conditioned taste aversion and is largely a nonconscious, instinctive alteration of the acceptability levels of particular food tastes if that flavor is associated with the onset of illness, nausea or pain. Although we can consciously teach ourselves to avoid particular foods that do not agree

with us, conditioned taste aversion at its most basic is noncognitive learning. Experiments have shown that animals have such reactions, even if the association of the taste stimulus and unpleasant consequence occurs under general anaesthesia. When our food preferences alter dramatically during illness, part of the alteration may well be an evolutionarily ancient and protective mechanism "attempting" to prevent us from contacting a possibly noxious food a second time.

In health and disease, in our conscious and unconscious existences, in ways we are scarcely aware of, our sense of taste is an abiding sampler of the chemical nature of the world around us. It is a sense which developed and was refined in a world of natural chemicals, but which still serves and protects us on a planet now pulsing with artificial molecules. Having charted the marvels and usefulness of this faculty, we are better able to understand the predicament of the sufferers from familial dysautonomia. This double recessive genetic condition, apparently restricted to the descendants of Ashkenazi Jews, leaves patients with a congenital absence of taste papillae. What a vital window on the world is forever closed to them.

101

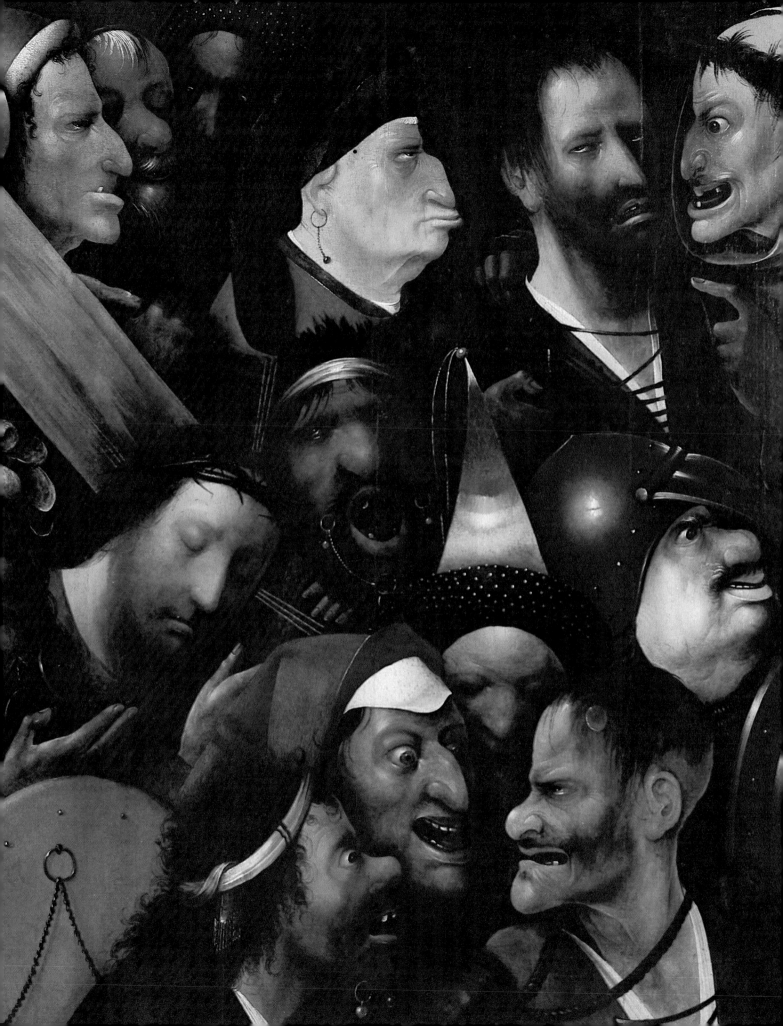

Chapter 6

The Mechanics of Smell

Historically, smell is the Cinderella of the senses. Until the time of the classical Greeks, there were no hard and fast ideas about the organ of smell, neither what it was, nor how it functioned, and even the Greeks were confused and inaccurate on the subject. Some of our modern understanding of the sense of smell, however, has its roots in the writings of Greek thinkers.

Democritus of Abdera (460–360 B.C.) was an Atomist, who thought that men smell things when atoms of various shapes, sizes and textures impinge upon the nose, producing qualities that trigger characteristic sensations. The famous philosopher Aristotle (384–322 B.C.) was not nearly so mechanistic. He believed in the doctrine of the four elements: that all things were composed of earth, air, fire and water in varying proportions and were further characterized by being hot or cold, moist or dry.

Aristotle thought that the sense of smell was largely to do with fire. He claimed that the organ of smell had to be cold — being so close to the body's cooling system, the brain — but was potentially hot. And, since the object of smell, an odor, was a hot, smoky exhalation, smelling was a matter of the organ of smell being warmed more or less.

Galen of Pergamum (A.D. 131–201) was a famous Greek physician and a most prolific writer, whose ideas about medicine and human biology went unchallenged until the Renaissance. Since he could not see any olfactory hairs in the nose, Galen thought that odors literally penetrated the olfactory bulb, which he rightly maintained was part of the brain. Here the odor was changed into cerebral pneuma, or winds — the *spiritus animalis* — and was carried to the brain's cavities.

He suggested that the brain pulsated rhythmically: when it contracted, it sucked the pneuma in, and when it expanded, it expelled the remaining pneuma. In addition, he thought that the olfactory bulb acted as the brain's excretory organ, which, when the brain expanded, discharged mucus into

Grotesque faces provide much of the drama of this savage painting, entitled Christ Carrying the Cross, *by Hieronymus Bosch. Since most of the faces are in profile, noses dominate the scene, their exaggerated shapes lending a malicious power to the expressions of Christ's tormentors. Modern cartoonists, too, find the nose the best feature for caricature, holding, as it does, the key to the character of many faces.*

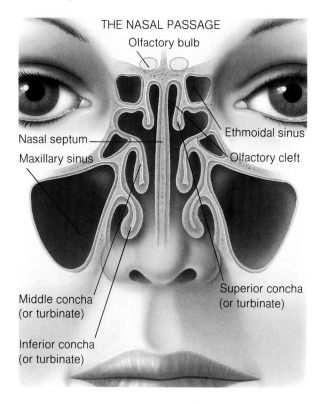

THE NASAL PASSAGE

Olfactory bulb

Nasal septum

Maxillary sinus

Ethmoidal sinus

Olfactory cleft

Middle concha
(or turbinate)

Inferior concha
(or turbinate)

Superior concha
(or turbinate)

the nose. Not until the seventeenth century was it realized that the source of the mucus was the blood serum and small glands.

In 1890, the Spanish neuro-atomist, Ramón y Cajal, unraveled the nerves and their main connections that led from the olfactory hairs, via the bulb, to the part of the brain associated with smell. Once Cajal and his successors had painstakingly sorted out the details of this pathway, there remained only two hurdles in the history of the study of smell. How do the molecules of an odor stimulate the sensitive cells of the olfactory membrane to produce a characteristic smell sensation, and how do the cells relay the resulting message to the olfactory center of the brain?

The Nasal Cavity
The part of the human nose that is concerned with smelling is surprisingly small and consists of two patches of yellowish-gray tissue no bigger than a postage stamp. These are located in a pair of clefts which lie just beneath the bridge of the nose, right at the top of the nasal cavity. About 95 percent of

the nasal cavity is quite unrelated to smells and smelling and is really an air-conditioning plant to clean and treat the air before it meets the sensitive and delicate tissues of the lungs.

The walls of the nasal cavity, and particularly the middle and inferior conchae (scroll-like bone flaps), are coated with unpigmented respiratory mucosa. This is provided with a vast army of tiny, hairlike cilia, which move wave after wave of mucus backward toward the throat. Bacteria, dust and chemical particles become entrapped in the sticky strings of mucus and are denatured — their properties are changed — by the stomach juices after the mucus is swallowed.

During normal breathing, only a tiny fraction of the air breathed in is able to penetrate the narrow entrance to the olfactory clefts. In fact, experiments have shown that airflow through the nose is characterized by great turbulence and many eddies and whirlpools. But when we sniff, the increased speed of air at the nostrils (perhaps three or four times the speed of 250 milliliters per second in normal breathing) causes a larger proportion of the air to travel high up into the cavity, and so to come into contact with the sensitive tissue.

When we have a cold, the production of mucus is many times higher than normal and may obstruct the narrow openings to the olfactory tissue. Under these conditions, which occur commonly, we become temporarily anosmic, or without a sense of smell. The shape of the upper part of the nasal cavity naturally varies from person to person, and some are more prone to nasal blockage than others. For some unknown reason, the exit passage from the back of the nasal cavity is larger in women than in men.

The olfactory membrane is slightly pigmented, but the function of the pigmentation is unknown. It has something to do with olfactory ability, however, because albino animals (which lack olfactory pigments as they do all other pigments) have no sense of smell. In parts of Virginia where redroot (*Lachnanthes tinctoria*) is common, farmers will rear only black pigs, since white (albino) pigs are regularly poisoned by eating the roots of this plant. White pigs cannot smell the plant and so are unprotected against eating it. Similarly in Tarentino, Italy, only black sheep are reared, since albinos are

Surrounded by notes on the study of grammar, this profile by Leonardo da Vinci is almost a caricature, the strongly marked nose and chin exaggerated and distorted in order to convey personality.

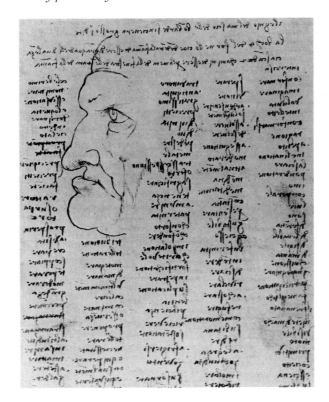

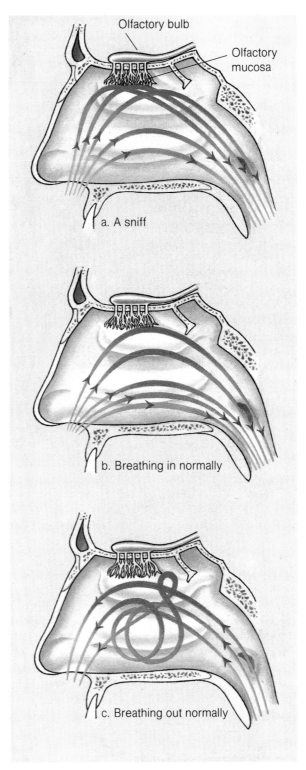

The flow of air through the nose while sniffing (a), breathing in normally (b) and breathing out normally (c), is shown in these three diagrams. When breathing normally, little air is forced up into the olfactory clefts, but during a sniff, when a person is deliberately trying to perceive odor, air currents travel upward to bombard the hairs of the olfactory mucosa, or membrane, with molecules of odor. Turbulent air flow typically accompanies breathing out, but enough air still reaches the olfactory mucosa to sustain perception of an odor.

Ramón y Cajal

Master of the Microscope

The eldest son of a respected surgeon in a remote village in the Spanish Pyrenees, Santiago Ramón y Cajal was wilful, rebellious and, what was worse, artistically inclined. Yet this boy, who pleased nobody, was to astound the academic world with his brilliant studies on the structure and function of nerve cells.

When he was sixteen, in 1868, Ramón y Cajal suddenly took his education seriously because his father allowed him to take drawing lessons. The world opened up for him; and he fervently studied natural history, chemistry and physics. Graduating in medicine from the University of Zaragoza in 1873, he spent two years in Cuba in the army. He then returned to his studies and, on passing an examination to teach anatomy, he wrote: "I aspired to be something, to emerge from the plane of mediocrity, and to collaborate, if my powers permitted, in the great work of scientific investigation that I hoped might bring some measure of glory to my sad country."

Ramón y Cajal became the source of the scientific renaissance in Spain. He also changed forever the course of neuro-anatomy and neurology.

While studying in Madrid in 1877, Cajal saw for the first

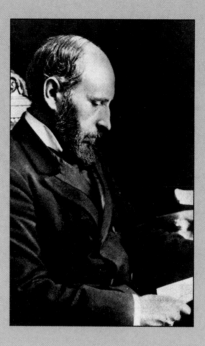

time the living world under a microscope; from then on, to whatever professorship he was posted, he devoted all his time to his microscope and to illustrating beautifully all that he saw through it. He was fascinated by the nerve cell, "... the aristocrat among the structures of the body, with its giant arms stretched out like the tentacles of a octopus to the provinces on the frontiers of the outside world, to watch for the constant ambushes of physical and chemical forces."

Cajal soon realized the value of suitable chemical dyes for staining the otherwise invisible structures he was seeking. He experimented with, and improved on, Golgi's silver stain and also used Paul Ehrlich's new methylene blue dye to reveal information about nerves.

So great was his expertise in histology that he made discoveries in all parts of the nervous system: he unraveled the nerves and their relationships in the olfactory bulb and lobes, the retina, the cerebellum, the medulla and the spinal nerves. Endowed with a special diligence and furious enthusiasm, he traced the intricate pathway of the olfactory nerves from the delicate receptor cells to the glomeruli in the bulb; and from the bulb to the complex neural network of the rhinencephalon, where he located the principal area of olfactory perception in the hippocampus.

Cajal is particularly famous for the proof he provided for one of the fundamentals of biological science—the neuron concept. He conceived neurons to be the basic units of the nervous system, which carry impulses in one direction only, from one neuron to another across tiny spatial gaps. For this work, in 1906, together with the great Italian histologist, Camillo Golgi, he was awarded the Nobel Prize for Physiology and Medicine.

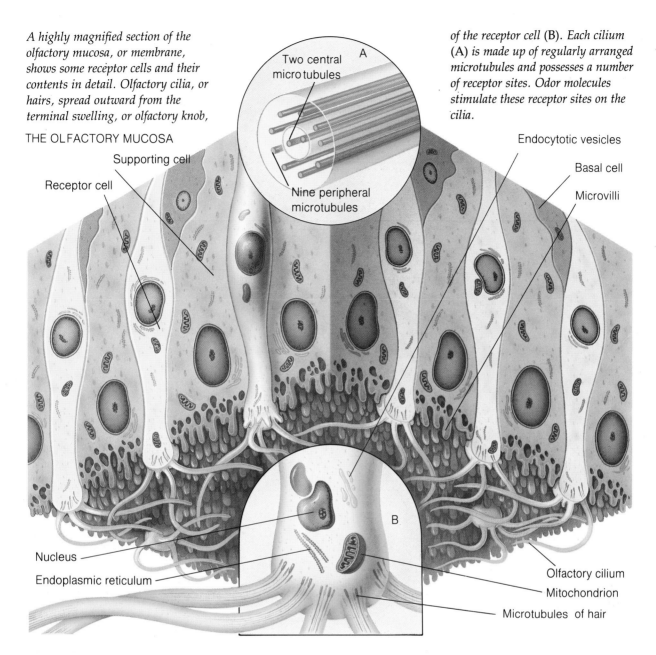

A highly magnified section of the olfactory mucosa, or membrane, shows some receptor cells and their contents in detail. Olfactory cilia, or hairs, spread outward from the terminal swelling, or olfactory knob,

of the receptor cell (B). Each cilium (A) is made up of regularly arranged microtubules and possesses a number of receptor sites. Odor molecules stimulate these receptor sites on the cilia.

THE OLFACTORY MUCOSA

A

Two central microtubules

Nine peripheral microtubules

Receptor cell

Supporting cell

Endocytotic vesicles

Basal cell

Microvilli

B

Nucleus

Endoplasmic reticulum

Olfactory cilium

Mitochondrion

Microtubules of hair

poisoned by eating St. John's wort (*Hypericum cristum*). Olfactory pigments appear to be of two kinds: carotenoids and free vitamin A, and phospholipids, but the whole question of their significance remains a puzzle.

Inside the Olfactory Membrane

The structure of the olfactory membrane is better understood. An electron microscope's view of the surface of the membrane resembles a plate of spaghetti in a viscous, or sticky, sauce. Each strand of spaghetti is actually a long, thin outgrowth from a small receptor cell. Each receptor cell, and there may be 10 million of them in humans, ends in a swelling, or olfactory knob, from which emanate

about five olfactory hairs. These are sometimes quite long, measuring up to one-hundredth of an inch, but most are much shorter. Where they touch their neighbors, there is often a slight swelling, as if the contact had produced some sort of new growth. The viscous "sauce" that bathes the whole membrane is mucus, produced from the basal regions of the membrane by glands known as Bowman's glands.

It is amazing to consider that these olfactory hairs are actually outwardly projecting extensions of the brain, which are in direct contact with the outside world, quite unprotected except for a thin layer of mucus about six-hundredths of a millimeter thick. The simplicity of this system, together with an

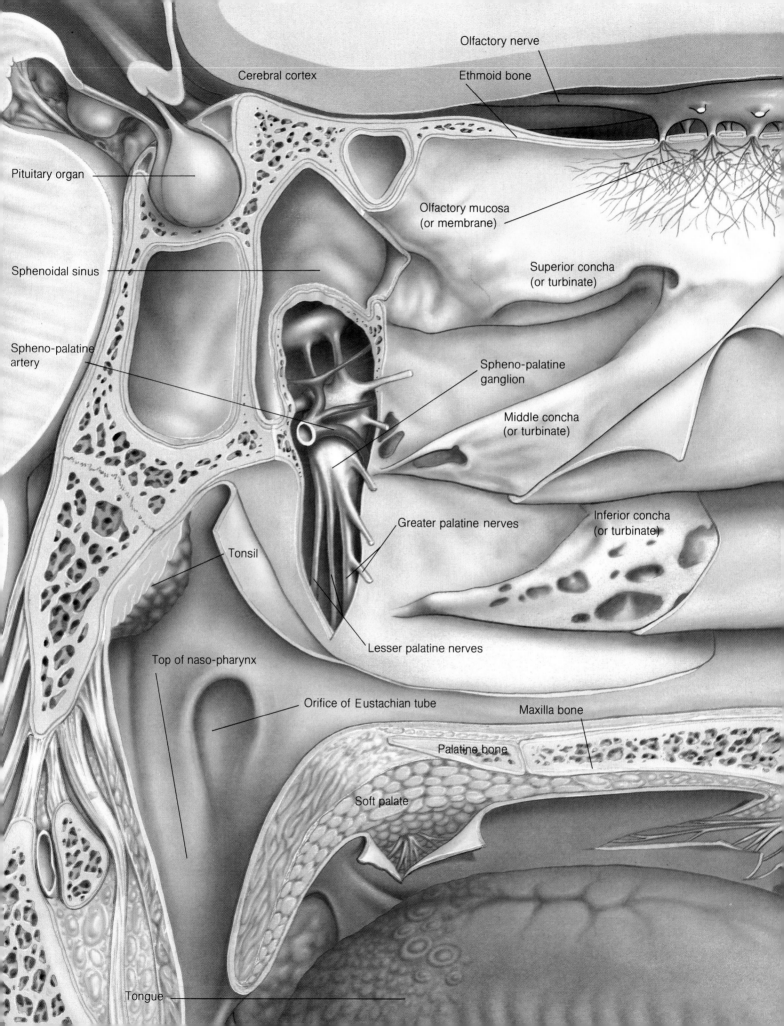

Olfactory nerve

Cerebral cortex

Ethmoid bone

Pituitary organ

Olfactory mucosa
(or membrane)

Sphenoidal sinus

Superior concha
(or turbinate)

Spheno-palatine
artery

Spheno-palatine
ganglion

Middle concha
(or turbinate)

Inferior concha
(or turbinate)

Greater palatine nerves

Tonsil

Top of naso-pharynx

Lesser palatine nerves

Orifice of Eustachian tube

Maxilla bone

Palatine bone

Soft palate

Tongue

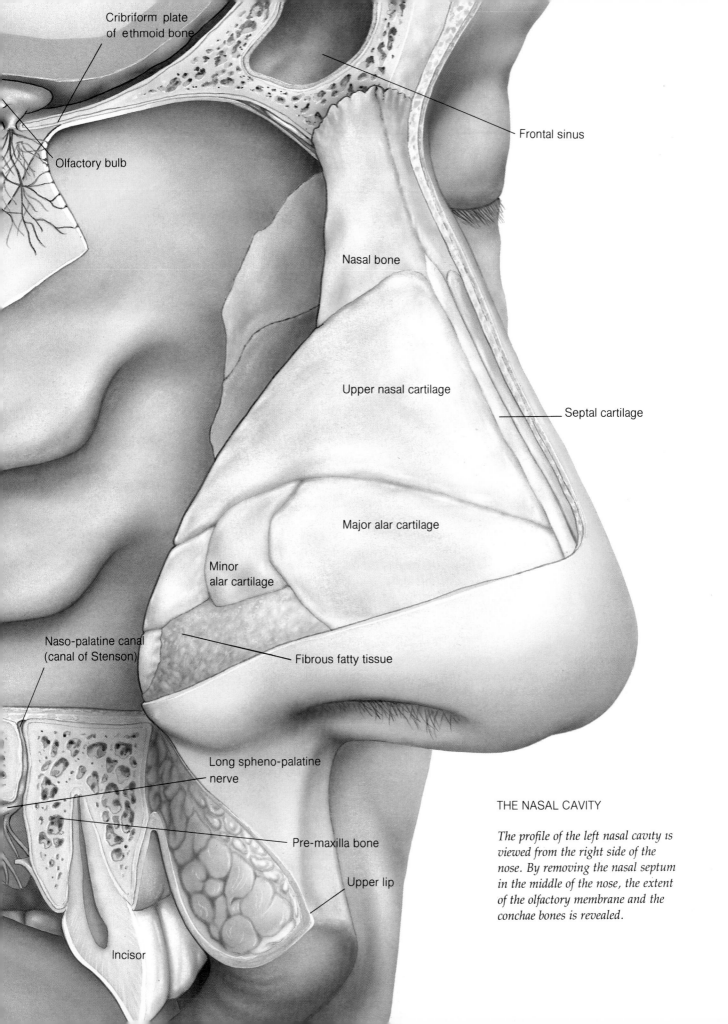

Cribriform plate
of ethmoid bone

Olfactory bulb

Frontal sinus

Nasal bone

Upper nasal cartilage

Septal cartilage

Major alar cartilage

Minor
alar cartilage

Naso-palatine canal
(canal of Stenson)

Fibrous fatty tissue

Long spheno-palatine
nerve

Pre-maxilla bone

Upper lip

Incisor

THE NASAL CAVITY

*The profile of the left nasal cavity is
viewed from the right side of the
nose. By removing the nasal septum
in the middle of the nose, the extent
of the olfactory membrane and the
conchae bones is revealed.*

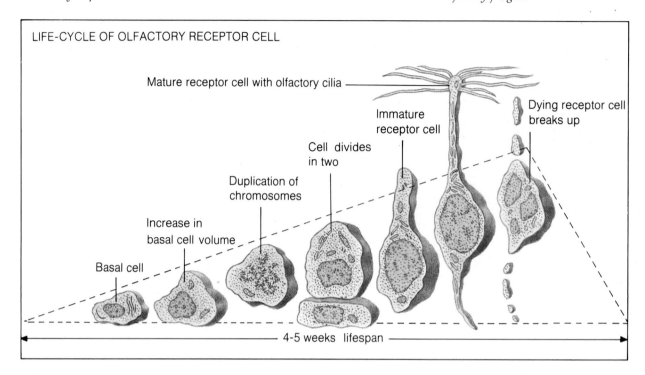

LIFE-CYCLE OF OLFACTORY RECEPTOR CELL

Mature receptor cell with olfactory cilia

Dying receptor cell breaks up

Immature receptor cell

Cell divides in two

Duplication of chromosomes

Increase in basal cell volume

Basal cell

4-5 weeks lifespan

extraordinary lack of structural variation of the olfactory receptor cells and hairs throughout the animal kingdom, suggests that the sense of smell is evolutionarily very ancient. By contrast, the light-receptive cells in the eye and the sound-receptive cells in the ear are hidden away from the outside world by a barricade of structures.

A price must be paid for this simplicity, however. Many cells become damaged, perhaps when the respiratory epithelium is overloaded and unable to execute its filtration duties effectively, so must be replaced. So, surprisingly for the nervous system, which is not renowned for its regenerative properties, there is a constant production of new receptor cells in the olfactory membrane. These grow from cells at the base of the membrane, thrust upward, become slender and sprout olfactory hairs.

In the mouse, it is known that each receptor cell functions for about twenty-eight days before it starts to break down and is removed by the mucus stream. Some researchers believe that another reason for this rapid turnover of cells is that the receptor cells actually absorb smells and must simply be discarded, like bags of household garbage, but this is by no means a universally held view.

In order to be able to begin to understand how the nose may work, it is necessary to know what an odor is. When we smell something, a stream of molecules from that object bombards the spaghetti-like surface of the olfactory membrane. Molecules are actually tiny particles, so it stands to reason that the lightest will travel farthest. Chemists have named this phenomenon volatility — the most volatile substances being those with the lightest molecules. Large, sluggish molecules, like those of candlewax, have far less smell than those of, say, violet petals or lavender.

Perceiving Odor

Odors are borne by the wind and air currents, as anyone who has spent time on open prairie land knows. Only when we happen to perceive a smell do we turn ourselves into the wind and then sniff, so as to force more air into our olfactory clefts. When we wish to enjoy or identify a smell, we do not fill our lungs in a single operation. Rather we sniff in short bursts with short pauses in between. Similarly, if we wish to savor the smell of a rose, we pass the bloom from side to side, exposing its fragrance first to one nostril and then to the other.

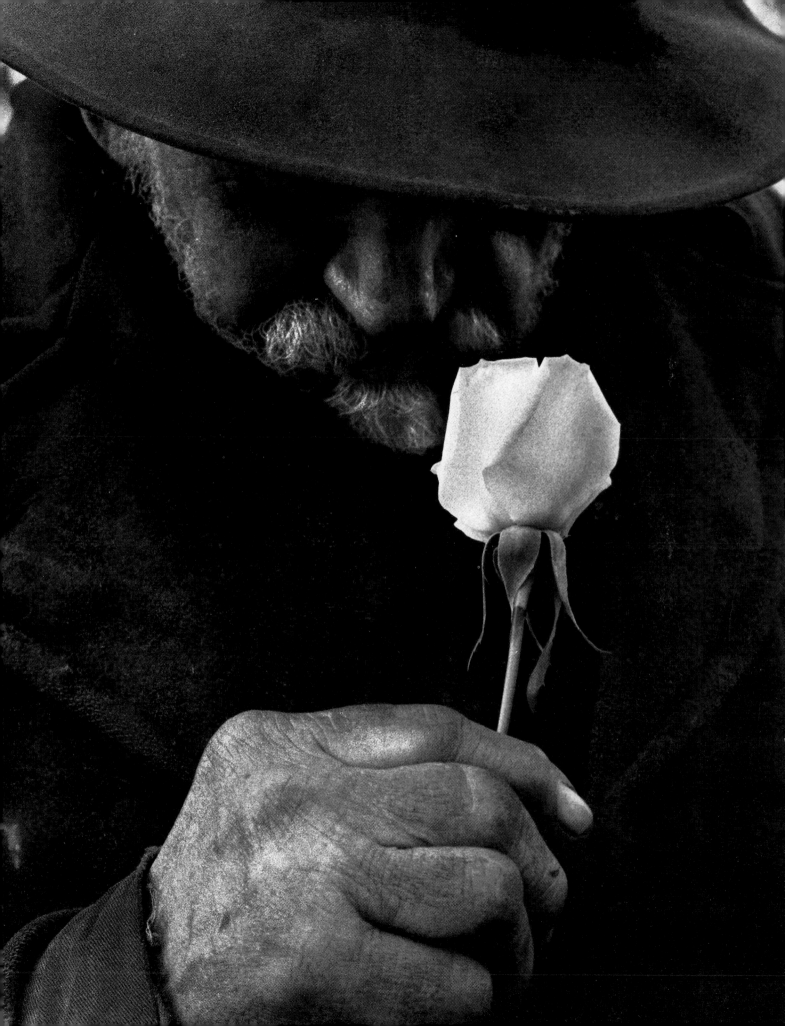

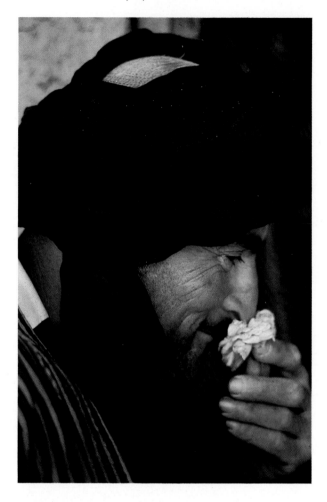

All this is to prevent odor fatigue, and in this respect the nose is very different from the ear and the eye. We can hear a particular pitch of sound for as long as that sound is made, and, if one sits in front of a certain picture in an art gallery, that vision will not change for as long as one stares at it. That is because both the ear and the eye rely upon units of energy to trigger them, and energy has no mass. The nose is not triggered by energy but by pieces of matter, which have a mass. Once a molecule has fired a response, it must be disposed of before a new molecule can trigger a new response, and that process takes a little time.

If the molecule comes along too quickly, there is no place for it on the olfactory hairs and so it cannot tell its story. If we watch a rabbit sniffing, we will see that it has a pair of flaps of skin which can alternately block off and open up the nostrils in a quick pattern of shut-open-shut-open. This avoids olfactory fatigue and enables the rabbit to keep in close odor contact with its environment. Everyone is sure to have noticed how a particular store, or friend's house, has a distinctive odor, which hits one on entering but which one becomes unaware of after just a few moments. This is because the nose is fatigued to that particular smell and no longer perceives it.

R. H. Wright, a physiologist from the University of British Columbia in Vancouver, suggests a simple experiment to try. Take a white and a red clover blossom. Both have a rather similar floral odor. If we sniff first the white and then immediately turn our attention to the red, the latter appears to have no smell. If we do the test the other way round, the red clover has a smell but so also does the white. It is almost as if the white clover has a few additional smell components, which we can perceive even when the odor of the red flower is still in our nostrils.

Tests such as this strongly suggest that there must be a number of specific sites on the olfactory hairs, onto or into which certain molecules stick or are absorbed. Here we experience one of the most fascinating aspects of modern medical physiology, for we simply do not know just how the nose works. A number of theories have been proposed, but none is yet universally accepted.

A basic problem is discerning which molecular quality has the capability of effecting a response. Molecules have a physical shape as well as an atomic composition. Many researchers have tried to show that the chemical (atomic) construction of the molecule gives it its smell, arguing that when a molecule hits a receptor cell hair, a number of chemical reactions take place as the molecule dissolves into its fatty outer surface. The quality of the odor depends upon the nature of these reactions and the rate at which they take place.

The Structure of Odor

But many problems remain, the main one being that chemically saturated compounds should not react as fiercely as unsaturated compounds and thus should have no smell. In general this is so, but the large family of saturated alkanes (methane,

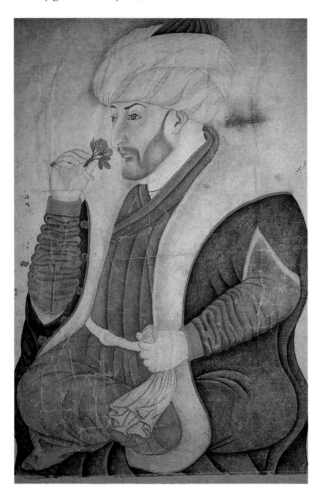

ethane, propane, etc) have rich, strong smells. Scientists today do not believe that the chemical composition of the molecule plays an important part in smell quality.

In the early part of this century, when science was much concerned with the electron theory in physics, a German scientist, Teudt, put forward a fundamental idea which has proved to be of major importance, although not in the way he intended. Professor Teudt stated that since odors were molecules, and molecules were made from atoms, odor quality was a property of molecular structure. When atoms come together to make a molecule, a number of electrons are shared, moving back and forth between atoms with a frequency characteristic of the particular molecule. Teudt believed that this electron vibration triggered the odor nerves.

This theory has certain attractions, particularly since we know that the ear is responsive to the actual frequency of the sound produced, and that the eye perceives different frequencies of light as different colors. But the problem is that there would appear to be no vibration-sensitive detectors on the receptor cells — in fact, as far as we know, there are no such sites visible by the electron microscope. The vibrational theory has some modern proponents, who have amassed considerable circumstantial evidence in its support, but much work remains yet to be done to convince the scientific world that this is how odors are perceived.

During the middle part of this century, as knowledge of the way in which nerves act increased, some scientists turned their attention to the way in which incoming odor molecules might bring about the depolarization and ionic exchange phenomena demonstrated to occur in all nerves. As an impulse travels along a nerve cell, potassium ions, or electrically charged potassium particles, inside the cell are pushed out, to be replaced by sodium ions, which enter to correct the ionic imbalance. Then, fairly quickly, the sodium ions are pumped back out, at which point the potassium ions slip back in and the cell is ready to convey the next impulse. A number of physiologists argued that this certainly must also occur in the triggering of an olfactory response, but the problem was to understand how an ionic exchange could occur.

In 1953, Dr. J. T. Davies of the Engineering Department at Birmingham University, England, proposed that when the odor molecule landed on the surface of the receptor cell, lipid (fatty) molecules in the surface attached themselves to the odor molecule and dragged it through the membrane and into the inside of the receptor cell. As it went, it tore a hole in the membrane, through which the potassium ions escaped to the outside and sodium ions flooded in. As the tear healed, the ionic relationships were reestablished, and the nerve impulse was on its way, leaving the odor molecule inside the cell.

Davies argued that small molecules, such as those of ether, would have to penetrate the membrane in a large aggregation in order to make a big enough tear. Large molecules, such as those of the foul-smelling Beta-ionone, could be smelled at far

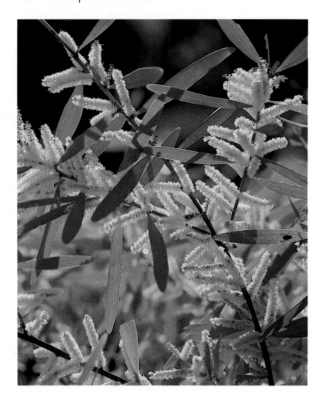

The development of X-ray diffraction crystallography following World War II enabled scientists to visualize the real shape of molecules. Professor Teudt, some five decades earlier, had suggested that the odor of a substance depended upon its molecular configuration, but he failed to take the importance of shape, or stereochemistry, into consideration.

Just as we have seen earlier with respect to the tongue, a minor change in a molecule's shape may prevent it from triggering a particular set of receptor points. It may even trigger a different set, in which case a different odor is perceived. It has been found that the most subtle change in molecular configuration may exert a powerful effect on odor quality.

Why Smells Smell

It would appear that there are a number of physical sites on the olfactory hairs into which odorant molecules can fit. This is a modern version of the ancient idea of Roman poet and philosopher Lucretius (*c.*90–55 B.C.) that foul-smelling substances have hooked and jagged particles, while sweet-smelling substances are made up of smooth pieces. Recently, in 1983, it has been shown that a class of synthetic molecules containing 16 carbon atoms smells like larger 20-carbon molecules. This is because of an inherent flexibility in the smaller molecules, allowing them to rotate into conformations that resemble the profiles of the larger molecules.

Of all the theories put forward to explain why smells smell, this one, involving molecular shape (stereochemistry), seems the most probable. It is true that receptor sites have not been shown by advanced electron microscopy, and neither do we know what happens to the molecule after it has plugged into its specific site. The answers to these questions will emerge in time, but we now have a working hypothesis that things smell as they do because of the shape of their molecules.

Mention was made earlier of the fact that the receptor cells were forward projections of the brain, protruding into the outside world. In fact, there is just a single cell running from the olfactory mucosa in the nose into a part of the brain called the olfactory bulb. In humans, this bulb is small — about the size of a matchhead — and it lies about four-tenths

lower concentrations because they were capable of causing a large tear on their own. Davies also argued that different receptor cell membranes would heal at different rates and that musks, for example, would stimulate only those cells with slow-healing membranes. By contrast, ether molecules, which are too weakly absorbed, would be unable to stimulate musk-sensitive cells.

The study of receptor cells with the electron microscope has failed to find any differences consistent with the idea that certain cells are responsive only to certain types of odor. Another difficulty with this "Penetration and Puncturing Theory," as it is called, is that sometimes an optical isomer (a mirror image) of a smelly molecule has no odor at all, yet is the same size.

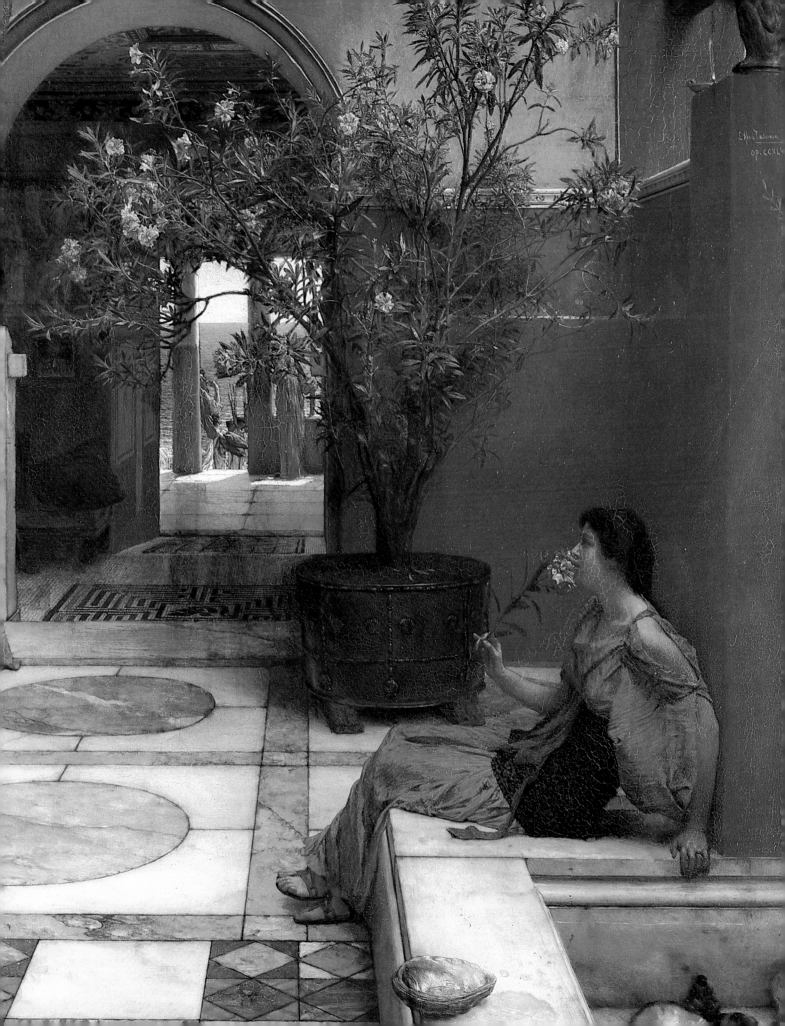

Odor signals go from the olfactory membrane to the olfactory bulb via nerve fibers. The primary neurone penetrates the cribriform plate and makes contact with the secondary neurone in the glomerulus.

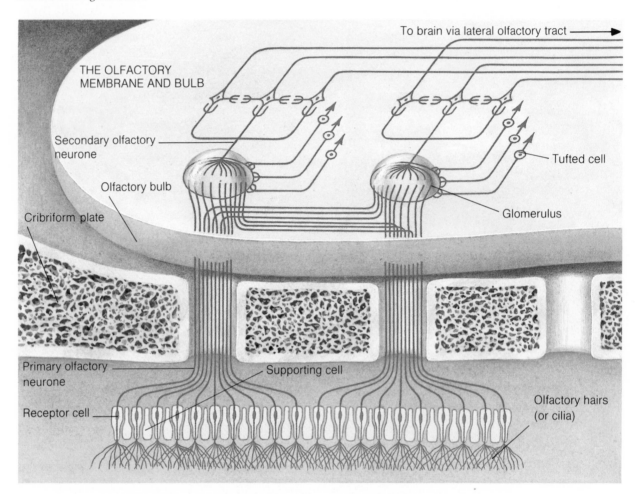

THE OLFACTORY MEMBRANE AND BULB

To brain via lateral olfactory tract →

Secondary olfactory neurone

Olfactory bulb

Cribriform plate

Tufted cell

Glomerulus

Primary olfactory neurone

Supporting cell

Receptor cell

Olfactory hairs (or cilia)

of an inch in and slightly downward from the bridge of the nose.

In order to reach the olfactory bulb, the axon, or large appendage from the receptor cell, has to pass through the cribriform plate, a small, penny-sized, sievelike patch of waferthin bone at the front of the cranial cavity. The olfactory bulb lies up against the cribriform plate, and, in the bulb, the cells make their first synapse (junction). This occurs in structures known as glomeruli, of which there are fewer than 2,000. This means that the 10 million or so receptor cells converge on just 2,000 glomeruli, which act as a series of telephone switchboards.

From each glomerulus there are two sets of output cells. First, there is a patch of twenty-four "tufted" cells that cross to the other olfactory lobe. Then there is a second batch, again of just twenty-four

cells, that form the second olfactory neurones, which continue their journey into the brain. Both the primary and secondary olfactory neurones lack the fatty white sheath of myelin associated with most nerves, as does the third neurone. Only when the fourth fiber takes over is a myelin sheath apparent. Unmyelinated fibers allow only a slow speed of neural transmission and are found mostly in invertebrate animals. Their persistence in the vertebrate nose is a further indication of the unchanged nature of the olfactory system throughout the eons of evolutionary time.

Little is known about the function of the glomeruli and why there should be such a reduction in the number of nerve fibers leaving them. But since each cell in each batch of twenty-four can be either "on" or "off" — nerve cells can never be only

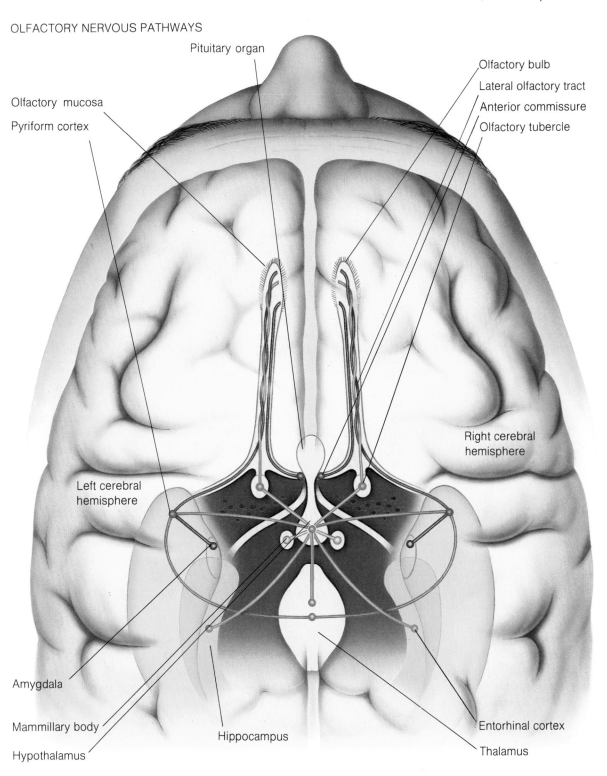

Most of the olfactory nerves that run from the olfactory membrane end in the center of the brain, which is evolutionarily the oldest part. But there are connections with the more modern cerebral hemispheres.

Pituitary organ

Olfactory bulb

Lateral olfactory tract

Anterior commissure

Olfactory tubercle

Olfactory mucosa

Pyriform cortex

Right cerebral hemisphere

Left cerebral hemisphere

Amygdala

Mammillary body

Hypothalamus

Hippocampus

Entorhinal cortex

Thalamus

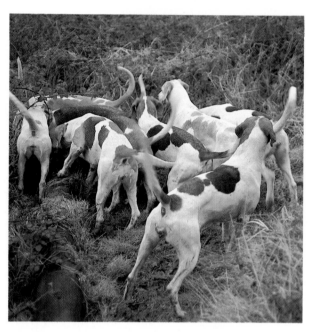

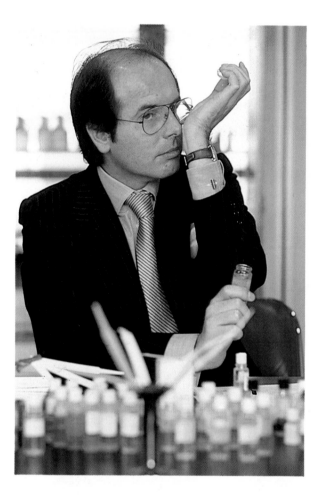

A perfumer in the famous house of Chanel samples a scent. Instead of simply sniffing at the bottle, he is testing the odor on the skin, since that is where it is to be used. The warmth and texture of the skin can subtly change the character of perfume, and this is what gives it individuality from wearer to wearer. A perfumer builds up a memory bank of different types of odor used in the making of scent and must be chemist as much as artist to know the way in which certain ingredients react with one another.

partly on or partly off — the number of permutations and combinations in this batch is something in the order of 16 million. If the quality of an odor is expressed by a certain pattern of "on-ness" and "off-ness" of cells in the batch, then theoretically we should be able to perceive 16 million odors. A trained perfumer, or tea or whisky blender, may need to use up to about 100,000 odors, so it would appear that in humans the system does not run at anywhere near full capacity.

After it leaves the glomerulus, the second olfactory nerve runs along one of the lateral olfactory tracts, synapsing with the third neurone in the region of the brain known as the amygdala. From here, the neurones penetrate to the basal and deeper regions of the brain, such as the thalamus, entorhinal cortex and the lateral and basal nuclei of the amygdala itself. An offshoot goes to the olfactory tubercle and on to the preoptic-hypothalamic region, the latter part of which region has connections with the pituitary organ. Thus the sense of smell has a direct access to many parts of the brain, unlike sight and hearing which are first processed by a relay center in the cerebral hemispheres.

Such a direct access is not surprising, considering the evolutionary antiquity of the sense of smell. Of particular interest is the way in which the olfactory

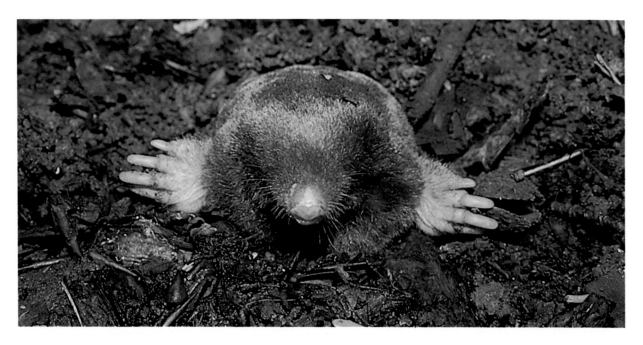

neurones make direct contact with the "oldest" parts of the brain—oldest in an evolutionary sense. These parts have relatively little to do with higher thought processes but are more closely identified with emotion and sexual behavior. Collectively, these parts are known as the limbic system (Latin *limbus* = a border), because they form the ringlike base to the massive cerebral hemispheres.

Taking the brain as a whole, only a minute part of it is devoted to the sense of smell. The paired olfactory lobes may even be overlooked because they lie tucked away at the base of the brain and are overlain by the cerebral outgrowths. In lower vertebrates, the olfactory lobes may be massive; in sharks they are the brain's most dominant feature.

Powers of Discrimination

It is a common misconception that humans have a poor sense of smell, but there are two facets to olfactory sensitivity — acuity and discrimination. It is true that we do not have a very acute sense of smell — odorants can be perceived only at fairly high concentrations. For example, the human threshold for acetic acid is about fifty million million molecules per cubic centimeter of air; for dogs it is half a million. Thus dogs perceive this rancid, sweaty odor at a concentration 100 million times lower than can man. Dogs have extremely acute noses and can perceive most odors at hundreds of thousands to hundreds of millions times lower concentrations than man.

It has been calculated that an average person sweats about 800 milliliters of sweat each day. Because of the dense aggregation of sweat glands on the soles of the feet, it is thought that as much as 2 percent, or 16 milliliters (half a fluid ounce), of sweat is produced by the feet each day. If as little as one-thousandth of this penetrates the soles and seams of shoes, it can be calculated that of an acid such as butyric acid at least as much as 250 thousand million molecules would be left behind in each footprint. As this is over a million times more concentrated than the dog's threshold for this odorant, tracking becomes child's play! Weather conditions and the type of ground influence the rate at which the scent evaporates, but trained dogs can usually pick up a trail up to twenty-four hours after it has been made.

Humans may not have an acute sense of smell, but their powers of discrimination are equal to any in the animal kingdom. People with trained noses, perfumers and the like, can distinguish between many thousands of odors and can retain a memory of them from one testing session to the next. The

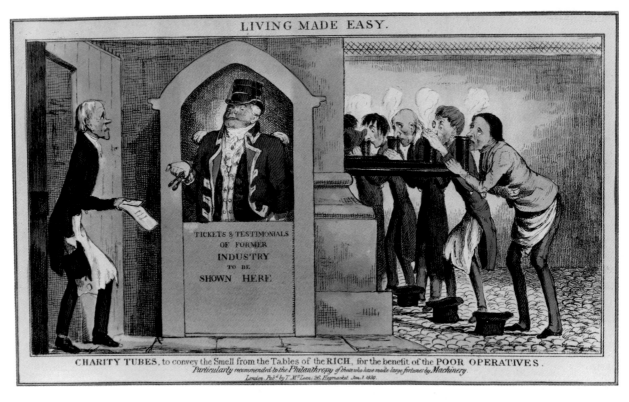

One of a series of comic suggestions for "Living made easy," published in 1830, shows skinny paupers inhaling the tantalizing smells of food from the rich man's house. A cruel joke, since nothing is more stimulating to the appetite than the aroma of good food. Equally, the smell of badly cooked, greasy food can be nauseating and extremely offensive to all but the sharpest hunger. Smell is an important part of our enjoyment of food. When sitting down to a delicious meal, the first action of most people is to sniff and appreciate its aroma. Such action has a base in fact: at one time the smell of food was a way of checking its freshness and suitability for eating. Spoiled food would be rejected because of its smell.

experts are no different from other people; we all have the ability to develop our powers of olfactory discrimination. Blind people do this quite subconsciously and can recognize visitors by the subtlest of odor clues. Since individual odor permeates clothes and bedding, it is not surprising to learn that blind laundry workers are able to identify even laundered garments and linen, when the levels of odorants must be vanishingly small.

Altered Sensitivities

There are many reasons why a person may lose his sense of smell, and temporary loss is a common phenomenon. A heavy cold has the effect of damping odor sensitivity by the overproduction of mucus and by the swelling of the nasal membranes. A specific infection of the olfactory membrane, known as rhinitis, may result in anosmia, or a total loss of smell. The same effect may stem from a number of allergies, all of which are associated with nasal congestion. Loss of the sense of smell may be associated with more serious conditions, however, such as tumors in the olfactory part of the brain.

Consultant rhinologists (doctors who specialize in the study of the nose) use a number of techniques to assess a patient's olfactory ability. All use one or another sort of olfactometry, a means of measuring ability to smell, in which the patient is presented with odors of gradually increasing concentrations, and it is his task to indicate at which concentration he first perceives the odor. The most often used odors conform to the seven major groups identified by physiologists who work on stereochemical research, that is, ethereal, camphoraceous, musky, floral, minty, pungent and putrid. The fact that each rhinologist has his own system (unlike ophthalmologists and otologists who use a standard armory of techniques to assess visual and hearing ability) is testament to the lack of interest shown in the sense of smell during the development of modern medicine.

An altered sensitivity to odors is commonly encountered, especially during pregnancy. Substances previously pleasant-smelling now become repugnant. The reason for this is unknown, but the body's changed hormonal state exerts an influence on the olfactory membrane, frequently causing it to swell. Nasal blockage is commonly associated with pregnancy. Altered odor perception also occurs in some brain disorders such as epilepsy.

It has long been known that a strong odor can end an epileptic seizure, but, in a few cases of the disease, a seizure is preceded by an olfactory hallucination, in which either an organic type of odor is hallucinated (putrefaction or decay) or a chemical one (ether, petroleum, chloroform). Only occasionally is it an agreeable odor. Some patients report altered sensitivity to odors for as long as a few days before a seizure. In some cases, normal odors such as food odors become unpleasant, and the subject feels unable to eat.

More rarely, the patient experiences a greatly enhanced sensitivity, often associated with abnormal feats of memory. This is known as the Marcel Proust syndrome, after the French novelist, who reported that certain odors brought back torrential floods of memory to him. Unusual sensitivity to odors, sometimes resulting in patients going to unnatural lengths to rid themselves of their own body odor, is commonly associated with schizophrenia type psychoses. All such neural disorders

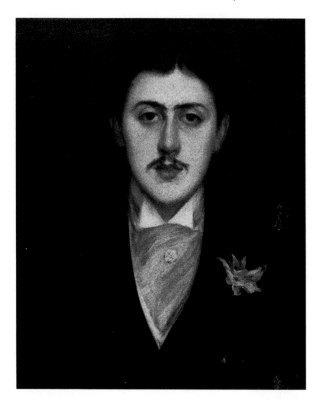

are rare, and the average person will live his life without ever experiencing more than the slightest disturbance to his sense of smell.

Before continuing to explore the world of odor in which we live, we must ask why we have a sense of smell at all. Nowadays, we can almost do without our sense of smell — with a heavy head cold, life continues much as it did before, although most people start to complain when food continues to lose its luster for long.

People's lives have been saved by their perceiving the odor of burning, or gas. (In Britain, where most domestic gas comes from the North Sea and is odorless, a smelly odorant — ethyl mercaptan — is introduced into the pipelines so that gas leaks can be detected.) Even recently, food was considered suitable for eating if it smelled good (pork is still subject to the sniff test in some places), and spoiled meat was rejected on account of its smell. But in our distant past, many aspects of our ancestors' lives were governed by the sense of smell, particularly sexual behavior and reproduction. These and other matters are dealt with in the next chapter.

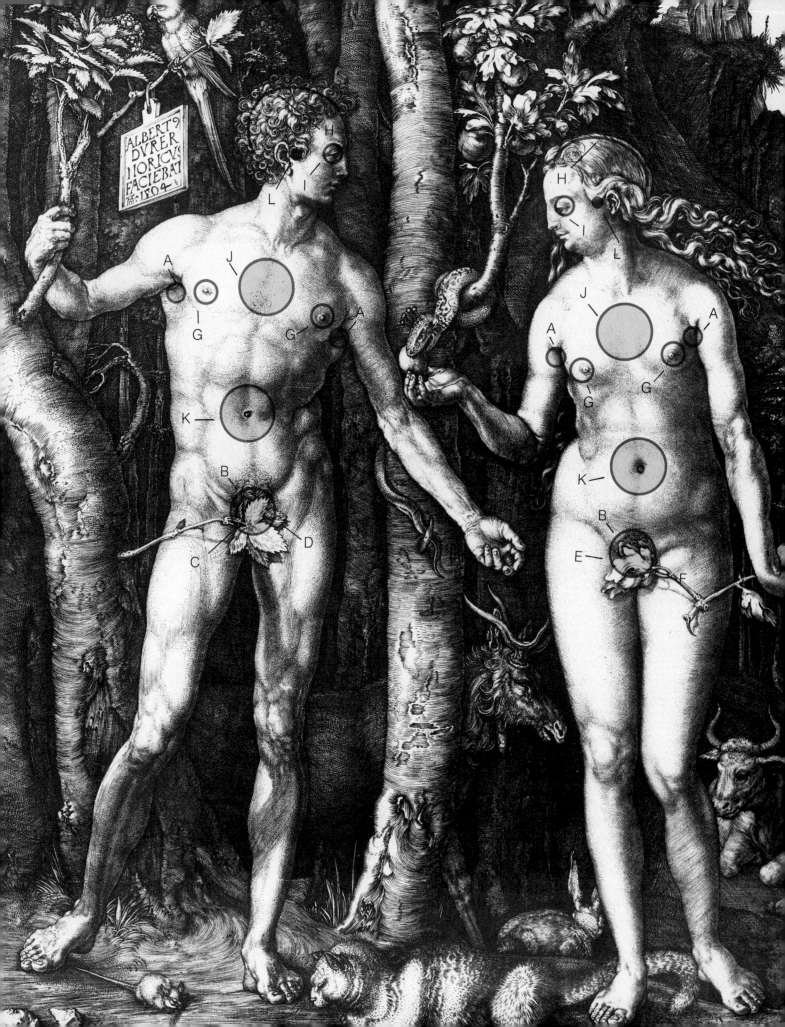

Chapter 7

Odor as Communication

Humans have a sense of smell which, while not being very acute, is far from redundant. Many lives have been saved by a sensitive nose picking up a whiff of smoke or poisonous vapor or detecting spoilage in food. But humans are remarkable in another olfactory context: they are astonishingly odorous. Nobody would argue that riding on a crowded subway in New York or Washington on a hot July evening is an odorless experience. Far from it, the stench of rancid sweat may be overpowering.

These smells, however, are not produced inside the body. Sweat is a colorless, watery and almost odorless fluid, which is pumped out onto the surface of the skin by the two million or so coiled sweat glands which lie deep within the dermis. Their secretion evaporates from the skin, cooling it as it does so. But the skin is host to countless millions of bacteria, which thrive in the warm, moist surroundings; and as they multiply, they produce metabolic waste products that consist of short-chain fatty acids, all of which smell more or less goatlike. Scrupulous attention to personal hygiene keeps the bacteria in check, and the use of antibiotic soaps keeps even the toughest sweat problem under control.

Glands in the Skin
But also lying in the skin are two other types of gland, both of which are associated with the hair follicles. First, each hair has its own sebaceous gland, producing sebum, whose primary function is to condition the hair, keeping it waterproof, oiled and free from other organisms that try to grow on it. Some people have overactive sebaceous glands and must wash their hair daily in order to prevent a rather smelly buildup. Second, the hairy parts of the body are richly endowed with apocrine glands, which are also associated with the hair follicle but are more like the sweat glands in structure. Both sebaceous and apocrine glands produce fatty

Superimposed on Albrecht Durer's engraving Adam and Eve, *are the areas of the human body that bear scent organs. The axillary organ in the armpit (A) is the most important of these, followed by the ano-genital region (B). Scent glands cover the scrotum (C) and root of the penis (D) in males, and the labia majora (E) and mons veneris (F) in females. There are also scent glands surrounding the nipples (G), on the scalp (H) and around the eyes (I). Blacks may have scent glands on the chest (J) and above and below the navel (K), while some Caucasian men have scent glands below the navel. Australian aboriginals are unique in having scent glands in front of the ears (L).*

Watery secretions of the sweat glands evaporate on the skin and cool a body overheated by physical exertion. Any odor is caused by bacteria on the skin, which multiply fast in the warm, moist sweat.

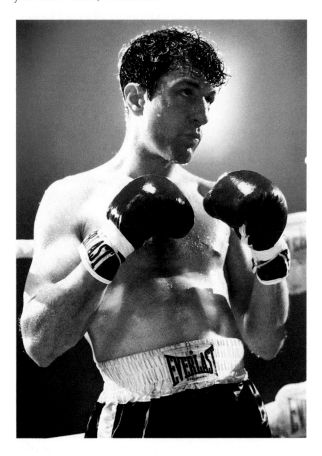

secretions; the difference between them is that each cell in the sebaceous gland breaks down, so cellular debris is mixed with sebum, while apocrine secretion is free from cellular material.

Sweat glands are fully formed at birth and start their activity immediately, but the true scent glands develop slowly during childhood to start their scent production at puberty. They continue to be active until the menopause in women, when the body's supply of hormones dries up, and they slowly decline in activity in men, in line with the gradual waning of male sex hormones.

The Scent Organ in the Armpit

As an ape, the human is noticeably hairless, although considerable thickets remain in a few places. By far the most important human scent organ is found in the armpit, or axilla as it is correctly called. An axillary organ occurs in both men and women and can measure up to just over one and a

quarter inches by half an inch. The springy hair that covers this region grows only at puberty, suggesting that the significance of the region is associated with sexual development. The secretion of the axillary organ is a mixture of watery sweat, which pours down the arm and chest, and a thick, yellow-brown oil, which tends to become tangled in the mat of hair. The secretion itself has a warm musky odor and is quite fragrant, but the waiting hordes of bacteria soon turn it into a goatlike stink. If this builds up, the concentrations of fatty acids reach such high levels that clothes may rot and skin allergies may develop.

Chemical Signals

Axillary organ odor has been closely investigated by scientists and has been found to contain steroid substances consisting of twenty carbon atoms arranged in four interlocking rings and belonging to the family of 16-androstenes. Steroids are used in the body in the production of sex hormones such as the female hormone, estrogen, and the male hormone, testosterone. Some steroids have strong odors to some people, and androstenol, a musky smelling androstene, can be readily perceived at concentrations as low as one ten-millionth of a gram at 68°F, when held four inches from the nose. A normal healthy man between eighteen and forty-five years old produces fifty times this amount from each armpit each day. Curiously, right-handed people produce about 75 percent of their total bodily output of axillary androstenol from the right armpit and left-handed people from the left armpit. Women generally produce only trace amounts of androstenes, but an occasional woman will produce levels more normally found in young men.

These 16-androstenes also occur in human urine. More occur in male than female urine, though the human testis does not make much of this steroid; by comparison, the pig produces vast amounts of 16-androstenes in the urine and in the saliva. It has been shown that sows are particularly sensitive to the odor of androstenol when they are approaching estrus (heat). One whiff of the substance and they adopt a rigid mating posture, with the back held straight and hind legs slightly apart, so pig breeders now use aerosol sprays of androstenol to detect which sows are ready for artificial insemination.

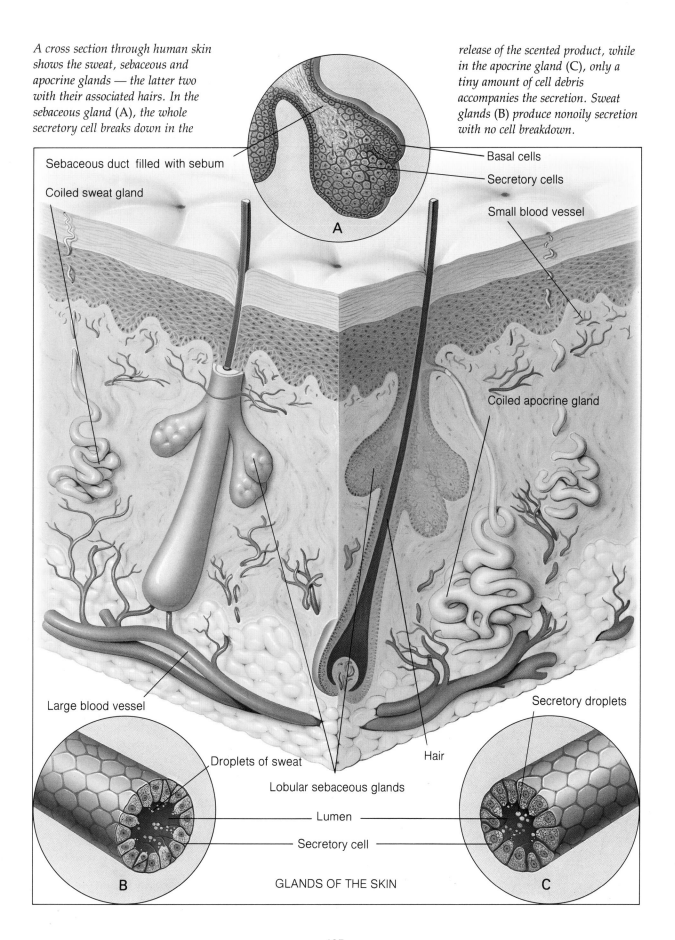

A cross section through human skin shows the sweat, sebaceous and apocrine glands — the latter two with their associated hairs. In the sebaceous gland (A), the whole secretory cell breaks down in the release of the scented product, while in the apocrine gland (C), only a tiny amount of cell debris accompanies the secretion. Sweat glands (B) produce nonoily secretion with no cell breakdown.

Sebaceous duct filled with sebum

Coiled sweat gland

Basal cells

Secretory cells

Small blood vessel

A

Coiled apocrine gland

Large blood vessel

Secretory droplets

Droplets of sweat

Lobular sebaceous glands

Hair

Lumen

Secretory cell

B

GLANDS OF THE SKIN

C

125

A zone of scent glands surrounds and covers the nipple of the female breast. The glands are associated with the milk ducts and odor is thought to be an important factor in the bonding of mother and child.

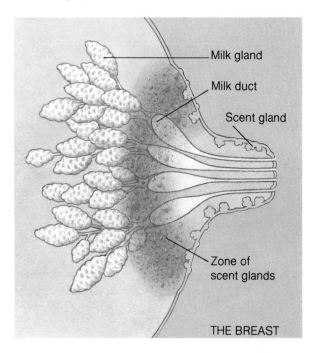

Milk gland

Milk duct

Scent gland

Zone of scent glands

THE BREAST

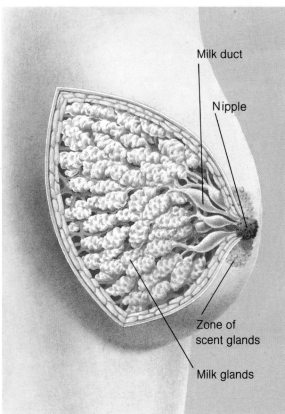

Milk duct

Nipple

Zone of scent glands

Milk glands

16-Androstenol is thus an example of what is called a pheromone — a chemical signal that passes from one individual to another and brings about either an internal physiological change or an observed behavior change. Insects have long been known to use pheromones to govern their sexual lives, but the progress of research in the mammalian field is slow. The existence of human pheromones is still a matter for debate but there is no reason why some aspects of human behavior should not be controlled by pheromones.

Areas of Odor

Why is the human armpit such an important source of odor? This region does not contain scent glands in any other species of mammal, with the exception of the chimpanzee and possibly the gorilla. The answer would appear to lie in the fact that humans walk upright, with their noses held high up above the ground. In much the same way as a dog lifts its leg to spray a jet of urine onto a post at roughly the height of a dog's head, so the area of olfactory interest in humans has moved up the body, away from the ano-genital region to the armpits.

The reason why the armpit rather than, say, the midline of the chest has developed as a scent organ is that in upright, bipedal man, the arms hang downward and cover the organs. Only when the arms are raised somewhat can the odor effectively escape. In this respect, the axillary organ of man functions like the scent-emitting organs of butterflies and moths, in which the odor source can be shut away when it is not required. No such control would be possible on the midline of the chest. It is significant also that the human female has well-developed scent glands on the breasts, which have been a sexual focus only since man adopted an upright stance and which, together with the axillary organs, are well positioned to allow a mutual perception of the odor of the other during the initial stages of courtship. This was delicately recognized and beautifully expressed by the early eighteenth-century English poet John Donne:

As the sweet sweat of roses in a still,
As that which from chaf'd Muskrat's pores doth trill,
And as th' Almighty Balm from th' early East,
Such are the sweat drops on my Mistris' breast.

(Elegie VIII)

126

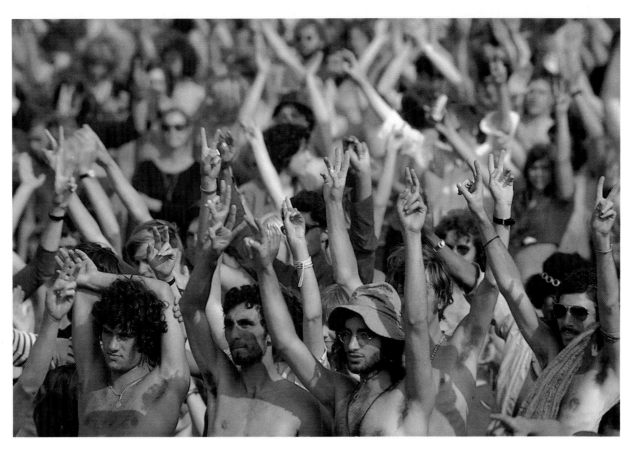

Before exploring farther the link between sex and the sense of smell, it is necessary to complete our survey of the location of human scent organs. Next in importance after the axillary region is the ano-genital region. A ring of scent glands surrounds the anus, some half an inch from it, and together with glands covering the scrotum and root of the penis in males and the labia majora and mons veneris in females, produces the characteristic odor of this area. The hairs that occur in the ano-genital region are, like those in the axillae, rough and springy and well suited to act as wicks. Little is known about the substances produced from these glands, but steroids are once again abundant. As we shall see later, ano-genital odors are significant to people suffering from various neuroses and psychoses. A few less-important areas are found to have scent glands, notably around the nipples in both sexes and on the scalp. Scent glands surround the eyes, pour their secretions into the tear ducts and from

there into the nose, to be disseminated during breathing. They are also found around the lips and the margin of the nose itself.

Racial Characteristics
The occurrence of scent glands is not uniform throughout mankind and certain races have their own characteristics. In some Blacks , scattered scent glands occur in the skin of the chest and on the abdomen, both above and below the navel. Caucasians have no chest glands, and only a tiny proportion of men have abdominal glands, which are always below the navel. Australian Aboriginals have scent glands in front of the ears, a position in which scent glands have been found in no other humans, and they also have an exceptionally well-developed anal organ, comparable in its function to the Caucasian's axillary organ. Mongolid people have extremely weakly developed scent glands, with the least scented being the Korean

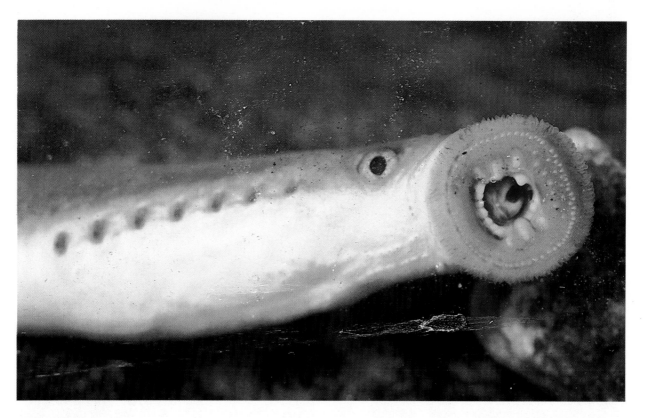

Huanghoids. In this group of people the axillary organ may be absent.

Mention was made above that the axillary organ of Orientals is but little developed. Indeed, until a few years ago, the possession of underarm odor was considered sufficient reason for a young man to be discharged from the Imperial Japanese Army. If the same rule applied to our own armed forces, there would be no armed forces!

Smell and Sexuality

Puberty in humans heralds the blooming of the body's odor garden. Glands develop under the influence of sex hormones, and hair grows to aid in odor diffusion. At this time we become aware of our own smell, and that of others, and adopt more rigorous hygiene procedures than before. This relationship between body odor and sexual maturation was recognized two thousand years ago by Aristotle, who observed that certain eunuchs lacked a sense of smell. Today we recognize a number of congenital defects affecting both the nose and the sexual system. One of the best known is Demorsier's olfacto-genital dysplasia, in which the olfactory lobes are not fully developed. Such people also show undeveloped ovaries and testes and have abnormally low levels of pituitary gonadrophic hormones, whose function is to cause the development of the gonads; sufferers are anosmic.

A similar situation is seen in Kohn's syndrome, in which abnormal development of the olfactory nerve is associated with undeveloped ovaries and testes. Again there is an impairment in the production of pituitary hormones. Is there a link, then, between the sense of smell and the pituitary-gonadal axis, which these phenomena would seem to suggest? To answer this, we must turn our attention to the lamprey, a primitive jawless fish.

The lamprey is held in special affection by anatomists because it represents an extremely primitive stage in the evolution of the vertebrate animals. It has large eggs, the development of which can be studied with ease in the laboratory. Early on in the development process, a small, slightly sunken disk develops on what is to be the front of the embryo. As the embryo grows, this disk sinks deeper and migrates upward and backward. Then a remarkable event occurs. One side of the disk dips down and pushes itself underneath the front of the developing brain. As the brain grows, a small vesicle (which was the edge of the disk) enlarges and adheres closely to the brain, but it does not lose its threadlike connection with the remainder of the disk, which now develops into a saclike organ at the side of the respiratory organ.

This sac subsequently becomes the olfactory organ (and the lamprey is unique in having just a single organ), while the part underneath the brain

128

becomes the anterior part of the pituitary organ — the part which produces the hormones that cause the ovary and testes to develop. Although details of the embryological relationship between the pituitary and the olfactory organs are more obscure in humans, the lesson from the lamprey shows us that there is an ancient link between the two systems in this most ancient of the senses.

The anterior part of the pituitary organ is well known for its hormone secretory function, but a point of which we must remind ourselves is that it serves another equally important function. It constantly has to monitor the levels of steroid hormones circulating in the blood, in order to integrate the hormonal orchestra of which it is the conductor. Our understanding of the olfactory–sexual link is facilitated by regarding the nose as a confrontational organ — an organ which, by perceiving steroid hormone output in the urine and body odors of others, confronts its own body's stage of internal readiness with that of others.

The Olfactory–Sexual Link

The link is very clearly seen in animals other than man, and the case of the pig has already been referred to. If the olfactory nerve of a rodent is surgically severed, the rodent shows no interest in courting a member of the opposite sex. In some species, for example the rat, this effect is seen only in sexually naive individuals. Once a rat has had sexual experience, its reliance on its nose for behavorial cues appears to be reduced. Other work has shown that exposure of a rodent to the odor of a partner of the opposite sex brings about a sharp increase in the levels of circulating steroid hormones. Humans now rely very little upon their noses for cues to control and regulate sexual behavior, though it would be wrong to suggest that odors play no part, as we shall see later on. So why has a primary reliance on odor cues been abandoned in favour of visual and acoustic ones?

The answer to this question is far from clear. The great Austrian psychologist Sigmund Freud argued that as man rose up from the ground his nose no longer was stimulated by earthly odors. Gradually, by a process of olfactory repression, he came to reject those odors, which before had helped him to survive. Freud does not tell us why man's ability to

use his nose should have become repressed, however. A possible answer may be found in a consideration of the social development of our species.

There was a time when our ancestors lived in small family groups, occupying the forest edge. Each group might have consisted of a single adult male, one or two adult females and their dependants. It was important that an estrus period — a period of ovulation — in the females would not be overlooked, and it would be advertised by estrous odors broadcast by the urine. Dr. Richard Michael and his team at Emory University, Atlanta, have demonstrated the importance of estrus-related odors in the mating behavior of the rhesus monkey. Similar cycles of odors are produced by women, and vaginal odor is said to be pleasant at the time of ovulation.

But when extensive prairie opened up in the Miocene epoch, some ten to twenty million years ago, a new sort of animal evolved — the large herbivorous ungulate. The presence of this rich food resource for the omnivorous (but quite strongly carnivorous) human ancestors provided a strong evolutionary pressure for behavioral changes to occur, which enabled small and puny man to kill large, horned herbivores. The result of this pressure was to cause a social change such that man now became gregarious, enabling cooperative hunting to occur.

Gregariousness, however, brought with it a new set of problems, for now it was possible for one particular female to attract a large number of males with her estrous odors, whereas before she could attract only one. The nuclear family was just as important within a larger communal group as it was before because it kept a single male bound to his females and, most importantly, his young. The period of juvenile dependence continued to increase as man evolved, so the patronage of a single male became more important.

It is wholly consistent with what is known of human evolution to postulate that olfactory repression evolved in order to preserve the bond within a nuclear family. The male would then be assured that one of his females was not unwittingly continuing to broadcast odor signals as to her state of sexual readiness. Gradually the repression became so rigorously fixed that humans could start to lift the lid of the repression just a tiny crack by the judicious use of perfume.

The decade immediately following the end of World War II was a most interesting one in almost every field of biology. The drug industry was becoming big business, and it demanded laboratory rodents in huge numbers for experimental processes. Animal husbandry suddenly developed, and much attention was paid to the biology of laboratory species. In Cambridge, England, Dr. Hilda Bruce made an observation of great significance. She noticed that if a recently mated female mouse was brought into contact with the odor of an adult male mouse (other than her stud male), her pregnancy was terminated and the tiny embryos resorbed. This effect became known as the Bruce effect, and was one of the first mammalian pheromone effects to be examined.

The Effects of Odor
At about the same time, two Dutch endocrinologists, Van der Lee and Boot, observed that if female mice were housed in quite dense aggregations, and, in the total absence of males, their regular four-day estrous cycles gradually lengthened until the females ceased to come into estrus at all. Many showed signs of pseudopregnancy. Just as Bruce had shown that anosmic female mice did not show pregnancy failure, Van der Lee and Boot showed that anosmic mice responded differently from controls. A few years later, Dr. W. Whitten from Bar Harbor, Maine, demonstrated that just the odor of an adult male mouse introduced to a group of females was sufficient to return all the lengthened cycles to a synchronous start, and a normal four-day cycle ensued. He showed that the odor responsible was in the urine, and that sexually immature or castrated males did not produce the necessary odor.

Since these three sets of observations were made, some twenty to twenty-five years ago, the total dependence of the mouse reproductive biology on odor signals has been carefully elucidated. This has led many biologists to ask whether there is any clear-cut evidence for the existence of human pheromones. After all, man has a reasonable sense of smell, at least in terms of discrimination, and a well-developed scent-production system. Is his repression so tight as to have precluded all pheromonal effects?

The first inkling that some effects may still occur came in 1971 from a study conducted among the occupants of an all-female residence, who were asked to record when their menstrual periods started and how much they mixed with men. It turned out that the degree of menstrual synchrony between room-mates was quite pronounced, and that the cycles of girls who saw little of the opposite sex were longer than those of girls who regularly spent time with men. On the surface, there appears to be a great similarity between human females and mice, but caution must be used in interpreting the results, since cycle lengths could be influenced by diet, work patterns and so on.

More recently, there has been at least one report of a young woman who noticed that each year at summer school her room-mates' menstrual cycles always synchronized with hers by the end of the summer. She was used in an experiment in which her axillary-organ secretion was collected daily on pads, and, after ether extraction, was applied to the upper lip of a group of female volunteers. A similar group received just a dab of ether, and nobody knew which group they were in. There was total asynchrony in the cycle starting-dates of the experimental group at the beginning of the experiment, and almost total synchrony five months later. Again the results must be interpreted cautiously, particularly since the size of the two treatment groups was small, but the implication is that there may be a pheromone in existence which is produced by females and which affects the reproductive cycle of other females. It would be interesting to know whether this "driver" woman has an unusually high level of axillary steroids.

Odor and Sexual Maturation
It is known from studies on mice that the onset of sexual maturation can be accelerated by submitting the young, prepubescent female to adult male odor. Dr. Alex Comfort, author of many books on sex and sexual behavior, has questioned whether the late onset of female sexual maturity in Victorian England was because young girls were kept in isolation from young boys and, among the upper classes, were even educated in private. He points to the

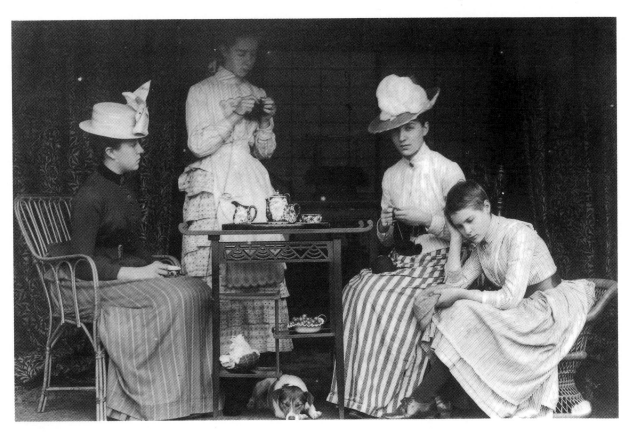

synchronization of the growth in coeducation with the fall in the age at which young girls start their periods and suggests that male odor, rather than nutrition, may be the causative factor. At the present time, there is much interest being shown in laboratories around the world in the possible existence of human pheromones. All the signs are that we should not have to wait long for some answers and that we may be amazed at what we learn. Our noses are far from non-essential.

Odor in Disease

Everybody knows what a normal, healthy human body smells like. Assuming it is clean and relatively free from surface-smelling bacteria, it smells quite pleasant. But in illness the odor changes dramatically. The characteristic sweet smell of acetone on the breath of a comatose patient should alert the doctor to diabetes, and parents should be on the lookout for this unmistakable odor in their children's bedrooms. Rubella, German measles, is reported to smell of freshly plucked feathers; in variola, chicken pox, the smell is said to be like that of a menagerie; in trench fever, like rotten straw. Experienced doctors can distinguish between the foul breath odor of Vincent's angina and the sweetish one of diphtheria. In some medical programs, students are being introduced to the odors of disease through "scratch and sniff" cards bearing microencapsulated chemicals.

The Odor Enigma

Thus it may be seen that humans are odorously extremely active. They produce huge quantities of odors from myriad sites in the skin, as well as in urine, feces, saliva and breath. And there is evidence that some fundamental physiological processes may be influenced by odors borne on the wind. Yet we have an obsession with body odor and spend millions of dollars a year removing it and, significantly, replacing it with a wide variety of expensive potions.

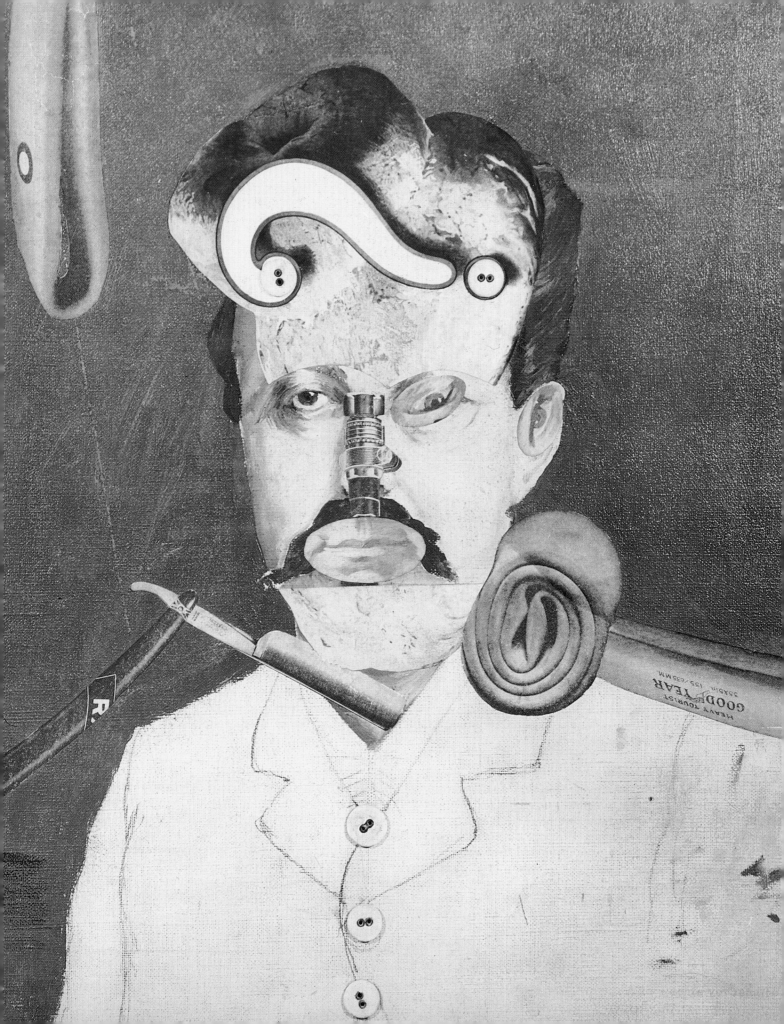

Chapter 8

The Enigma of Smell

No matter how good our sense of smell may be in discriminating between different odors, it cannot be said that this sense is a leading channel of intellectual curiosity. Many people would regard their sense of smell as being pretty nearly redundant, regarding human odor as being, in a sense, unclean and not worthy of civilized man. This is a curious aspect of our regard for our own noses. Smells are associated with tribal man and men less "civilized" than ourselves; we come to expect that the nose will be strongly stimulated by tribal customs and dwellings. For the average American housewife to be told that she, her family or her home smells of people would be a humiliating insult of the most serious nature. Yet humans are people. Why should there be such unease over this delicate subject?

The past twenty years have seen the two great, socially taboo subjects of sex and death come into the open for close scrutiny. We have learned to take a detached view of these matters, so we can stand back a little and view them from a new, almost clinical perspective. Why can we not do this with our own bodily odors? This is the fascinating enigma of the human sense of smell.

A Dispensable Sense?

If you were to stop a sample of, say, a hundred ordinary human beings on a busy downtown sidewalk and ask them which one of their five senses — sight, touch, hearing, taste and smell — they would be prepared to part with, were that necessary, just about everyone would choose their sense of smell. Some might be uncertain as to whether to choose taste, but would probably argue that never again to be able to taste a juicy apple or a well-grilled steak would be far worse than never being able to smell these foodstuffs. Also, they would likely say that they lose their sense of smell whenever they get a cold, but that life continues pretty much as before.

German artist George Grosz, 1893–1959, brought vitriolic social criticism of the materialism and hypocrisy of the twentieth-century world to his work. In the painting Remember Uncle Auguste the Unhappy Inventor, *Grosz merges the man and his technology, replacing the senses with the trappings of modern life.*

133

Despite the feminine image of scent advertising, men, too, have decided preferences, liking odors such as pine, lavender and violet. Violet was particularly popular with the Romans — men as well as women.

Look at these popular household goods. All promise to make the home smell of something else, such as lemon or pine, and these smells have now become synonymous in our minds with freshness and hygiene.

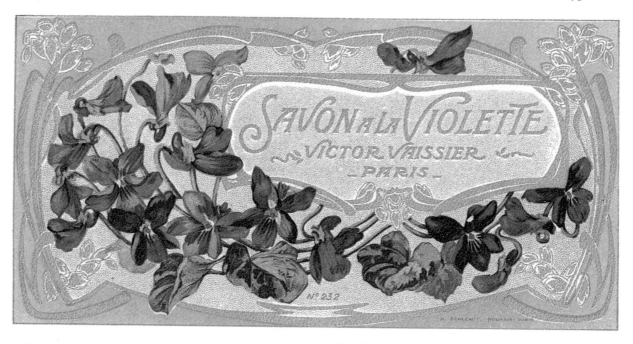

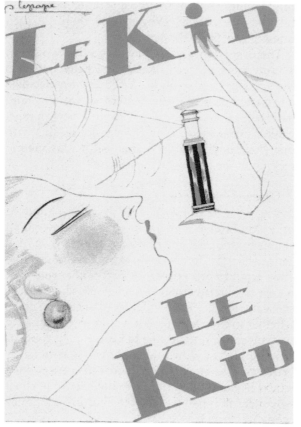

But if you were to ask these people a second question, you might be surprised at the answer. If you asked them whether or not in the past twelve months they had given or received a scented product, such as soap, perfume, aftershave or scented hair spray, practically everybody would admit they had. They would talk about these smells with open frankness, perhaps telling you that such and such a perfume goes rancid on them, but another retains its fragrance. Our civilized and hardworking housewife does not want her home to smell of its inhabitants, but she does want it to smell. She buys polishes and detergents and cleaning fluids, all of which contain extract of pine forests, wide-open prairies and Old English gardens.

Here is the nub of the enigma. We would part with our sense of smell more readily than any other sense, yet our lives are totally dominated by what we smell like. A fundamental tenet of our modern civilization is that odors are eliminated; a paradoxical tenet is that we have a powerful urge to appear fragrant to our fellow beings.

The author Somerset Maugham mused on this in his travel writings. The following extract from *On a Chinese Screen* illustrates his view of the relationship between smell and society: "When I lay in my bed I asked myself why in the despotic East there

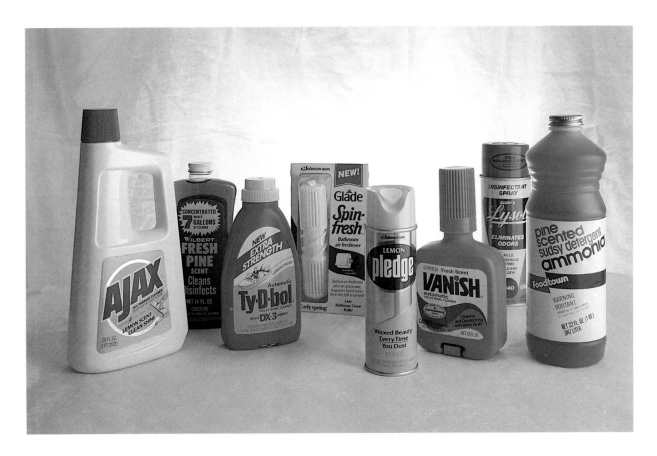

should be between men an equality so much greater than in the free and democratic West, and was forced to the conclusion that the explanation must be sought in the cess-pool. For in the West we are divided from our fellows by our sense of smell. The working man is our master, inclined to rule us with an iron hand, but it cannot be denied that he stinks: none can wonder at it, for a bath at dawn when you have to hurry to your work before the factory bell rings is no pleasant thing, nor does heavy labour tend to sweetness; and you do not change your linen more than you can help when the week's washing must be done by a sharp-tongued wife . . . . Now, the Chinese live all their lives in the proximity of very nasty smells. They do not notice them. Their nostrils are blunted to the odours that assail the Europeans and so they can move on an equal footing with the tiller of the soil, the coolie, and the artisan. I venture to think that the cess-pool is more necessary to democracy than parliamentary institutions. The invention of the 'sanitary convenience' has destroyed the sense of equality in men. It is responsible for class hatred much more than monopoly of capital in the hands of the few. It is a tragic thought that the first man who pulled the plug of a water-closet, with that negligent gesture rang the knell of democracy.''

Smell is not quite like our other senses. Its antiquity and pedigree give it a right to enter the innermost retreats of the mind, in which are locked away the ghosts and spirits of our evolutionary past, ever ready to pounce and remind us that we are, after all the pretense and posturing is stripped away, just animals. We are scared by what it might reveal in us if we try and view it with detachment. Our olfactory memory traces are an Achilles' heel, a soft spot overlying the very key to our personalities, which, for some quite inexplicable reason, natural selection has failed to patch. This is the reason for our unease. We recognize the central and fundamental role of the sense of smell in the basis of the psyche, and we know it to be a constant reminder of our animal origin. Civilization puts a distance between us, as humans, and the rest of creation. But, like an umbilicus, our sense of smell binds us fairly and squarely to all the other creatures on the earth.

The First Sensation

The moment we are born, we have to start breathing, and, if the first breath is not drawn within a minute or so of birth, brain damage may occur. Irrespective of where the human baby is born — in a dark mud hut or in a shiny modern hospital — the sense of smell starts its lifework within the

When a newborn baby is put straight to its mother's breast, its first sensory experience is of the scent glands surrounding the nipple. Smell is thus one of the baby's first clues for recognition.

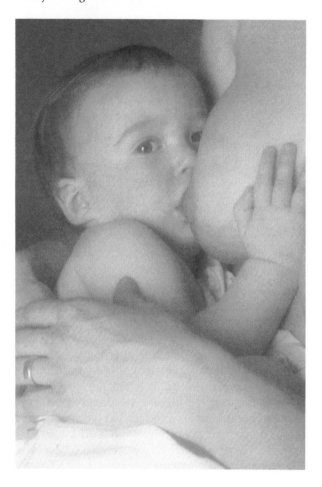

first few seconds of independent existence. Nowadays in modern hospitals, some newborn babies are put immediately to the mother's breast, where the nose nuzzles up against the bank of scent glands surrounding the nipple. The first sensory contact with the outside world, and the first and most abidingly familiar sensation the infant has, is an olfactory experience. The infant quickly becomes "imprinted" to its mother's odor.

We can only imagine what psychological damage is inflicted on infants who are removed from their mothers at birth (ostensibly to allow their mothers to rest) and are then fed milk from a bottle which lacks human odor, for little is known about the long-term significance of olfactory imprinting in humans. Dr. Michael Russell, from Sonora State Hospital in California, has shown that by six weeks of age babies respond much more positively to a

breast pad worn by their mothers than to pads worn by other lactating women, although it is unknown as yet to what extent milk and sebaceous gland odors interact.

The English psychologist Joan Fitzherbert has questioned whether bottle-fed babies are equally responsive to odors in later life as breast-fed babies, who are exposed to pleasurable odors immediately after birth. There is no doubt, however, that the sense of smell may be involved in pleasurable sensations in young children. Writing about severely disturbed and psychotic children, Dr. Fitzherbert notes that many lack either painful or pleasurable sensations from outside in both the emotional and physical spheres. Their only sensory perception is through smell, and she quotes an experienced teacher of such children who regularly noted that, when she changed her brand of toilet soap, the children sniffed her on and off for most of the day. It seems that imprinting must be pleasurable — the infant must recognize its mother as the source of all that is secure in its tiny world.

The Odor Bond

We do not know for how long olfactory imprinting occurs. In some animals it is known to occur very quickly, notably in goats. If a newborn kid is exposed to its mother for even a few seconds and is then removed, the mother will reject all other kids offered to it and accept its own kid after the passage of several hours. If the kid is removed before the mother has had a chance to sniff it, or if the mother has had its olfactory nerves surgically severed, the mother will likely accept a succession of strange kids and show no particular attachment to its own.

A short period for the establishment of this relationship is seen in sheep, too, and shepherds tell many stories of how they try to foster an orphaned lamb onto a ewe that has lost her own lamb. The most effective, if somewhat gruesome, way for this to be achieved is for the shepherd to skin the dead lamb and tie the pelt to the orphan, like a loose overcoat. At first suspicious, the bereaved ewe gradually comes to accept the orphan, and after a few days the often flyblown overcoat may be removed.

As the baby grows into a young child, his odor preferences begin to change. As a toddler, he is fascinated by fecal odor and sometimes appears bewildered when told by grownups that feces are nasty and should be disposed of quickly. It has been suggested that fecal and anal gland odor is a pronounced component of adult odor, and that the infant's pleasure in this keeps him close to his mother and prevents him wandering off.

Age and Odor Preference

It has been shown in rats that a lactating female, eleven days after littering, begins to produce a maternal pheromone in her feces that her pups find most attractive. At eleven days, rat pups are very alert, being fully furred and well coordinated. The likelihood of their wandering away from the nest at this age, and away from safety, is high. The production of maternal pheromone continues until the twenty-seventh day of lactation, which is when weaning occurs and the pups are encouraged to leave the nest.

Adult rats, like adult humans, are not attracted to fecal odor, though it is unknown whether they are as disgusted by it as are humans. As we saw before, disgust at the odor of feces and putrefaction has a survival value, for such materials are the source of life-endangering organisms. Freud has written much about the significance of the anal phase in a child's development; perhaps its retention in modern man is to assist the development of a bond between the child and his mother at a stage in the child's development when he may start to stray from his mother's side.

Young children are particularly fond of sweet, fruity smells, such as that of strawberries, and have little regard for heavy oriental odors such as musks. They also have less strongly held views about smells which adults find nauseating. When tested with a strong, but unfamiliar, odor, children younger than ten years old perceived it at slightly lower concentrations than adolescents, and at greatly lower concentrations than adults of twenty-one to thirty-nine years of age.

The fondness for sweet, fruity odors wanes around adolescence, when both boys and girls become attracted to heavy, oily odors of musk, sandalwood and patchouli. It is not only the manufacturers of candies who are aware of the odor preferences of preadolescent children; the recent

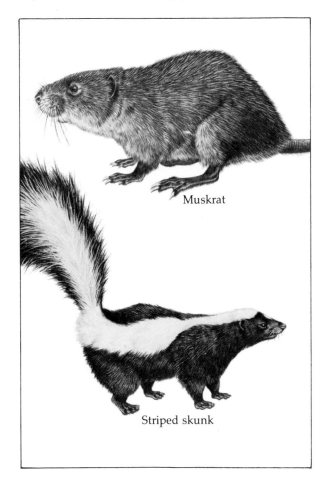

Muskrat

Striped skunk

appearance of pineapple- and strawberry-flavored erasers, pencils and various novelties is based on a careful interpretation of the known smell preferences of children.

In his classic work on human scent preferences, Dr. R. W. Moncrieff demonstrated that musk, which is a constituent of the sexual attractant odors of many species of animals and plants, becomes quite attractive to both girls and boys aged around fifteen. At about twenty years old, the attractiveness wanes considerably, only to rise sharply thereafter. Men over twenty-five are more attracted to the odor of musk than are women of the same age, but this difference gradually disappears with increasing age.

Human body odor changes markedly throughout life. In one of the *Claudia* books, the writer Rosa Franken comments that at about four years of age

Hendrik Zwaardemaker

Pioneer of Smell

They haven't got no noses,
The fallen sons of Eve.
And even the smell of Roses
Is not what they supposes.

G. K. Chesterton's witty rhyme underlines the problem facing any physiologist wishing to unravel the secrets of smell. The first man really to tackle the problem was an erudite Dutchman, Hendrik Zwaardemaker. Born in Haarlem, Holland, in 1857, he trained in the medical sciences, especially physiology and the study of the ear, but his most important work was the study of odors and our perception of them.

Zwaardemaker became internationally renowned when his book, *The Physiology of Smell*, was published in 1895 while he was teaching at the University of Utrecht. This book marked the beginning of scientific study of the human perception of odors.

He describes the experiments carried out of the olfaction sensations of a large number of people who differed widely in sex, age and status. For these experiments he invented a disarmingly simple device called the olfactometer. Each person sniffed and inhaled through a nozzle, a measured amount of a variety of odors. Using the olfactometer,

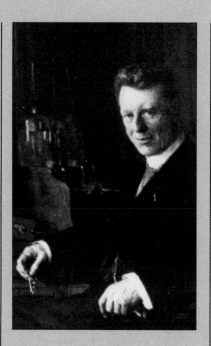

Zwaardemaker measured the minimum quantity of an odorant needed for the subject to detect it.

Zwaardemaker introduced two important concepts to the study of olfaction: adaptation and compensation. He found that the nose adapts to particular odors, so more and more of the odor is needed before its smell will register. He also found that if two similar odorants are smelled one after the other, far more of the second odor is needed than if it were smelled alone. Compensation occurs when certain pairs of odors, inhaled simultaneously through a

double olfactometer, reduce each other's apparent strength. Sometimes the odors in a pair compensate each other entirely, producing no smell. In the same book, the Dutchman makes his other contribution to the study of smell — a classification system that organizes all known odors into nine classes:

Ethereal: fruit, beeswax
Aromatic: almonds, clover, camphor
Fragrant: vanilla, balsam, flowers
Ambrosial: amber, musk
Alliaceous: onion, garlic, iodine
Empyreumatic: roasted coffee, tobacco smoke
Caprilic: cheese, sweat, goats
Repulsive: narcotics, nightshade
Nauseating: carrion, feces

Zwaardemaker supposed the odors of the first four classes to be pleasant, the last four to be unpleasant, while alliaceous odors are pleasant to some but not to others.

This classification system, assembled from several eighteenth-century taxonomies — most notably that of Carl Linnaeus, the famous botanist — and his own experiments, had a great influence on olfactory thinking in the first half of the twentieth century.

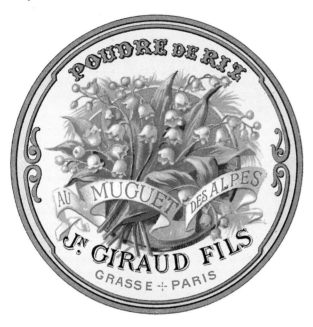

her heroine's young son ceases to smell like a baby and has the distinct smell of a boy. Baby smell is universally regarded as pleasant, especially by the mother, who will often inhale the odor plume emanating from the crown of her baby's head while the infant is being cuddled. The biological significance of an odor pleasant to the mother is not hard to understand. As was mentioned in the last chapter, the body's apocrine and sebaceous glands start to work in earnest when sexual maturity sets in, and at this time young people of both sexes cast aside their juvenile odors for ever.

It is interesting to note here that young European wood mice of both sexes smell much like their mothers until they become sexually mature, when the males quickly come to smell like their fathers. This system affords them protection in their prepubertal days from attack by adult males, who cannot distinguish them from females. When the young males are sexually mature, they must leave the nest and are immediately in competition with all other adult males for a territory. It behooves them to reflect their adult status in the olfactory as well as in the sexual manner.

A characteristic of human development is that it is very slow. Youngsters are not fully mature until they are eighteen or more years old. They may be sexually mature long before this, but mental and intellectual maturity develops more gradually. Natural selection and evolution have ensured that in most cultures the pair bond between the parents remains intact for as long as the children are dependent so that they may learn the skills of life from both parents.

Modern psychologists now believe that the eventual expression of the young person's sexuality depends upon a number of influences in the child's early life, although there is no doubt that the sex of human children is fundamentally determined at the moment of conception, when an X- or Y-bearing sperm fuses with the X-bearing egg. It is perhaps not surprising to learn that odor plays as important a role in human psychosexual development as it does in sexual attraction in adulthood.

Odor and the Oedipus Complex

A quarter of a century ago, the famous American psychologist Dr. Irving Bieber deduced from an analysis of olfactory hallucinations that odor played a role in what is called the Oedipal part of sexual development; that is, at the point where the capacity to react with sexual excitation to a heterosexual object is achieved. (This part of psychosexual development is named after the Greek, Oedipus, who, on solving the riddle of the Theban Sphinx, lost all human reason and married his own mother.)

Bieber argued that the onset of heterosexual reactions ushers in the Oedipus complex sometime between the second and fifth years, and that this response must be altered by a sensory procedure, which must, consequently, undergo a major change at this time. It is well known that at about five years of age young children's olfactory likes and dislikes change dramatically, one of these changes being the disgust shown to formerly attractive odors.

As can probably be appreciated, it is extremely difficult to gather details about the start of heterosexual reaction in humans because it occurs at a stage in life when the subject is hardly able to log and record his thoughts and emotions. One remarkable study exists, however, which centered on a little boy aged around four years old. He was an alert and articulate youngster, able to relate his feelings with surprising clarity. He also had a remarkably sensitive nose. From about his fourth birthday, he started to be repelled by his father's odor and, in particular, his axillary organ odor, though his head and hair smell was also involved in the repulsion. At the same time, the child would regularly cuddle his mother, and, when asked about the specific role of smell in his reaction, exchanges such as this took place:

Father: "What's the matter, Jackie, don't you like to hold Daddy close?"
Jackie: "I like to hold you close but not *too* close."
Father: "And how about Mommy?"
Jackie: "Oh, I like to hold her *very* close."

Dr. Michael Kalogerakis, a noted New York psychologist, who reported these observations, suggests that this differentiation in response to mother and father may be a part of the boy's growing sense of identity as a male. The boy was clearly repelled by male axillary gland odor which, it will be recalled, is first produced at puberty and contains sex steroids. It is, thus, the embodiment of the sex of the individual, and it is to this that the little boy reacted. It was stated earlier that the nose can be regarded as an organ with which the inner environment of one individual confronts the inner environment of another. This would appear to be as true for the young child as for the mature adult.

A feature of our modern times is that an increasing number of young children nowadays grow up in single-parent households, in which they are subjected only to the regular effect of the odor of either a man or a woman. It is as impossible to say what the long-term psychological effects of this may be as it is to say what are the effects of bottle-feeding. It would not be surprising if it turned out that these were significant effects.

The influence of the odorous environment on the growth and sexual development of mice has been the subject of much research. Young female mice show delayed sexual maturation when reared in a female-only environment, an effect which is negated if adult males, or just the urine of adult males, is present. Such experiments may be criticized for being highly artificial, for mice never occur in single-sex colonies. It could, perhaps, also be said that any disturbance in the normal pattern of human development resulting from a childhood spent in a single-parent family would be negated by the complexity of social contacts most young children make at school and at camp. The possible effects of odor deprivation on children from single-parent families is a facet of this modern phenomenon that has not yet attracted the attention of psychologists.

Smell and the Neuroses

There can be little doubt that our reaction to smells changes markedly at about five years of age. Prior to that age, the child derives a great pleasure from his sense of smell — Sigmund Freud called this "Riechlust." Freud was the first psychologist to ask if the Riechlust played any part in the genesis of the neuroses.

In his fascinating paper on compulsion neuroses, he says: "In a general way I should like to raise the question whether the inevitable stunting of the sense of smell as a result of man's turning away from the earth, and the organic repression of the smell-pleasure produced by it, does not largely share in his predisposition to nervous diseases. It would thus furnish an explanation for the fact that with the advance of civilization it is precisely the sexual life which must become the victim of repression. For we have long known what an intimate relation exists in the animal organization between the sexual impulse and the olfactory organ."

We saw in the last chapter why repression of the sense of smell was a necessary corollary of early humans adopting a gregarious life. (Interestingly, Freud himself gave no explanation for the repression of the sense of smell, a truly strange omission in such comprehensive writings.) What evidence is there that repression of Riechlust might play a part in man's predisposition to nervous disease? In his authoritative and extensive writings on the psychology of sex, Havelock Ellis states: "Many eminent alienists in various countries are of the opinion that there is a special tendency to the association of olfactory hallucinations with sexual manifestations."

For some reason, modern psychiatrists are not concerned with the sense of smell. There is abundant evidence relating to hysterical blindness, deafness, aches and pains, disturbances of locomotion, and hallucinations of hearing and sight, but few

*The association between sense of
smell and sexuality is proved, and,
in the same way that flowers attract
pollinating insects by scent, humans
use scents to make themselves
pleasing to others.*

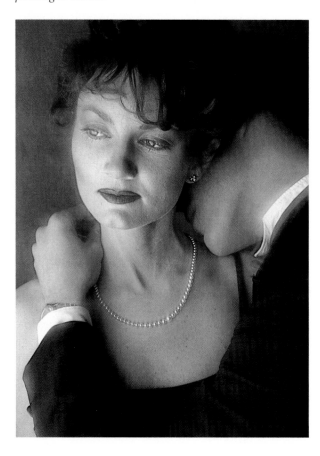

accounts of psychic disturbances of smell. Yet a few psychiatrists have recorded numerous examples of the central role played by smell in the neuroses and psychoses.

The famous American psychiatrist A. A. Brill records a case of a young man who was extremely sensitive to human body odors, particularly to female odors. His sexual behavior and reactions depended entirely on odorous sensations of the correct type. If a woman had any odor recalling his mother, he immediately became totally impotent in that woman's presence. An intelligent and resourceful man, he devised his own solution to this problem. He carried a bottle of perfume with him with which he liberally doused the woman in question in order to mask any odor of hers which he could link to his mother. By adopting this somewhat unusual remedy he was able to keep his particular odor neurosis under control.

Professor Brill writes about a number of patients

for whom Riechlust did not decline at the normal time and who retained an unnatural interest in fecal odor and that of sweaty feet. He hints that shoe fetishism, as the interest in feet is called, may be commoner than is thought. Such patients retain into adult life a great desire for smell gratification and they are often unable to make successful heterosexual liaisons. Many can be helped to live a normal life by seeking employment in a perfume factory or store, or in a florist's business, where the level of smell gratification is especially high.

Healing Odors

People with manic or schizoid-manic tendencies sometimes have hallucinations of odor, which dominate their psychoses, and the same has been observed in paranoids. Their dreams frequently involve odors — usually disagreeable ones — in one sexual context or another. There is no doubt that these unfortunate people have retained into adult life an interest in odors that normally disappears in childhood, and, in this respect, it may be said they have an olfactory capability similar to that of animals. Treatment of such cases is difficult, but attention to olfactory gratification is a therapeutic practice which may prove helpful.

Odor therapy is a new and little-tried means of bringing about behavioral change, but it is likely to be developed further in future. Considerable advances in this field have been made at the Sexual Behavior Laboratory at Atascadero State Hospital in California. In one study in this laboratory, a sexual sadist, who indulged in violent sexual intercourse, was subjected to a program of odor aversion therapy. His treatment was as follows.

As he was shown slides of sadistically stimulating situations, he was simultaneously forced to breathe in the odor of valerian, or garden heliotrope. This strongly scented herb produces valeric acid, which has, to most people, a fetid, nauseating odor. After several weeks of treatment, the patient's sexual arousal to formerly stimulating pictures was reduced to practically zero. Eight months after the treatment had stopped, his deviant response had increased only slightly. Since odor aversion therapy requires little in the way of complex apparatus and is ethically more agreeable than electric shock therapy, it is likely that we shall

A million rose petals are needed to make one pound of rose attar, or essential oil. The flower diagram, below, shows a generalized plan of suitable perfumes according to age, role and coloring.

The aromatic lavender likes stony ground and sunshine and, though a European plant, now grows well in California. Dried lavender has been used since Roman times, for both its aromatic and medicinal properties.

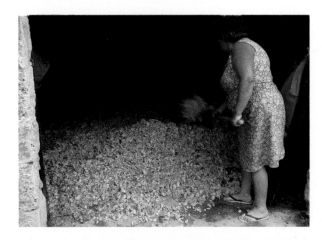

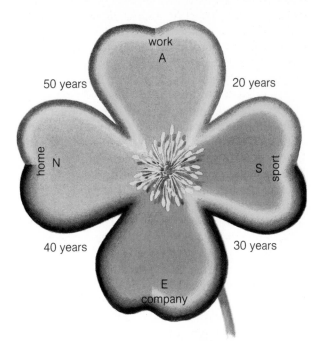

A = anti erotic (orange oil, lemon oil)
S = stimulating (oakmoss, patchouli oil)
E = erotic (jasmin, musk)
N = narcotic (rose)
A-S = fresh (spices)
S-E = exciting (castoreum)
E-N = sultry (amber)
N-A = soothing (bergamot oil)

- mother
- lover
- blonde hair
- red hair
- brown hair
- black hair

Read the above "flower" for each element independently.

see a rapid development of its potential for the treatment of certain types of psychotic patients.

The Emotional Link

The deep-seated relationship between perfume and the emotions has often been alluded to in the writings of Baudelaire, Tolstoi, Shelley and Wilde. In *The Picture of Dorian Gray*, Oscar Wilde gives this account of the influence of odor on the emotions: "And so he would now study perfumes and the secrets of their manufacture, distilling heavily scented oils, and burning odorous gums from the East. He saw that there was no mood of the mind that had not its counterpart in the sensuous life, and set himself to discover their true relations, wondering what there was in frankincense that made one mystical, and in ambergris that stirred one's passions, and in violets that woke the memory of dead romances, and in musk that troubled the brain, and in champak that stained the imagination; and seeking often to elaborate a real psychology of perfumes, and to estimate the several influences of sweet-smelling roots, and scented pollen-laden flowers, or aromatic balms, and of dark and fragrant woods, of spikenard that sickens, of hovenia that makes men mad, and of aloes that are said to be able to expel melancholy from the soul."

Certainly, perfumes mean more to their wearer and to others whom they meet than do the sight of fine clothes or the sound of soft music. In some way, which is undoubtedly related to the human suppression of interest in sexual odors, perfumes are provocative and revealing in a manner that sights and sounds can never be. During the course of human evolution, a point came when interest in sexual odors became so suppressed that it was quite safe for the memory traces of them to be stimulated just a little, and, from then on, perfumes entered everybody's lives. But how and why did the first perfume arise?

Origins of Perfume

There is no way we can answer this question with a high level of accuracy, but we can conjecture. It would not be unreasonable to suppose that, in the early days of gregarious living, women tended to gather fruits and berries while men hunted. An

142

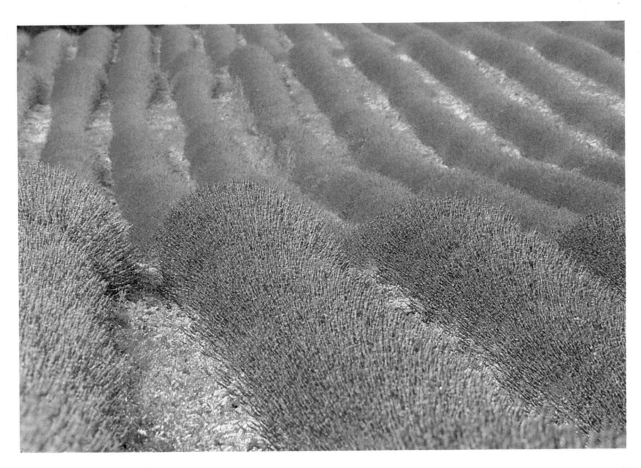

inevitable consequence of this was that women would become smeared with the juice and pulp of what they were gathering. Unconsciously, the first perfume had been born.

Nowadays we would call it a deodorant, because what it did was to mask the sexual odors. We can imagine that women better protected against unwanted sexual interest by males other than their established mates would be favored by natural selection over other women. As well as being protected, they were also, presumably, better fruit-pickers, and this would assist in their selection. Gradually, the use of fruit and leaf odors would have become culturally acquired, running in parallel with the gradual process of odor repression. Perhaps the use of perfumes as deodorants was just as important as repression of Riechlust in establishing the gregarious nature of the human species. In any event, after the repression was tightly enforced by natural selection, perfumes could be used to manipulate the mind.

Knowledge of perfumes extends back to the earliest times of recorded history and touches on medicine, mythology, religion and anthropology. The earliest recipes for the formulation of perfumes relied heavily upon what today we recognize as incense ingredients. Modern perfumes contain many essential oils of plants, that is, oily extracts from the odorous parts of flowers and from leaves and resins. The first essential oil to be distilled was turpentine from the terebinth tree, in the fifth or fourth century B.C., but it was not until the writings of the Spanish physician Arnaldo de Vilanova, in 1240, that we first learn any descriptions of essential oils and their production.

From the fall of Rome until the Renaissance, the development of perfumery was carried out mainly by the Arabs and Persians. The process they used to extract plant odors is called *enfleurage*. Flower petals were pressed between blocks of sheep fat or lard, into which the essential oil dissolved. Commonly jasmine, orange blossom and lilies were used to make a greasy pomade, which was then applied to the skin.

The use of alcohol to dissolve the essential oils of plants was not discovered until the fourteenth century, and the first toilet water was based on rosemary and called "Hungary Water." During the Renaissance, the center of perfumery moved to Italy and France, finally settling in Grasse, which overlooks huge fields of the finest lavender. In 1725, Eau de Cologne was first produced; it was

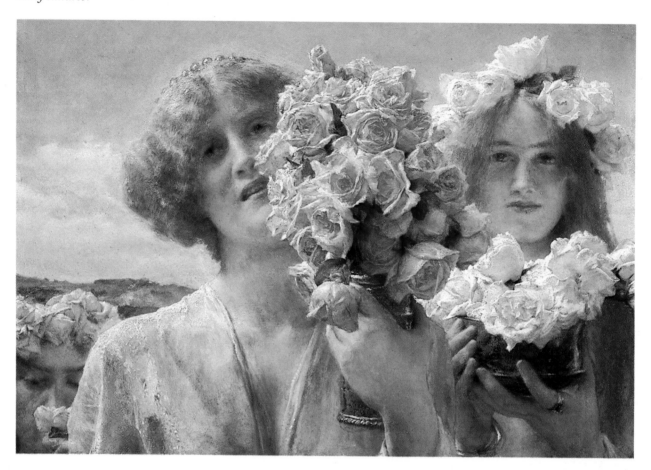

made mostly of a dilute extract of flower water of oranges. It was invented by the Duchess of Neroli, and even today is often known simply as neroli.

There have been many fashions in perfume since the Renaissance, the accent sometimes being on heavy floral notes (isoamyl salicilate and methyl-nonylacetaldehyde) or light, green notes (phanyl methylcarbinylacetate). But from the earliest times, animal sex-attractants have been mixed with perfumes. There are four main animal ingredients added to perfumes. They are musk, from the preputial pouch of the Oriental musk deer; castoreum, from the anal glands of the beaver; civet, from the inguinal, or groin, glands of the civet cat, and ambergris, from the stomach of the sperm whale. This latter is not a sex-attractant and appears to be a substance produced by the whale's stomach in response to scratching and irritation from the beaks of its chief prey — giant squid.

Musk, castoreum and civet are undoubtedly used in the overt sexual behavior of their producers, and their incorporation in floral perfumes considerably enhances the "mystique" of the fragrance. We use the word mystique here to make it clear that, subconsciously, we know that these ingredients are exciting to us, but we cannot say where the excitement comes from. Perfume manufacturers play hard on the subtle nature of the excitement by naming their creations "Shocking" (Schiaparelli 1935), "Tabu" (Dana 1931), "Je Reviens" (Worth 1932), "Intimate" (Revlon 1955). Some of these perfumes are now half a century old and are still being prepared to the original recipes.

Recently, a range of perfumes has been launched which contains androstenol — the steroid substance that in pigs acts as a mating pheromone and which is also produced in the axillary organ of man. To many people, androstenol has a distinctly urinary odor, and many professional perfumers know that, to be really successful, a fine perfume must contain a urinary note. Whether the addition of androstenol to the perfume markedly enhances its erotic effect is open to question.

In parts of the Austrian Tyrol, however, it used to be the fashion for young men, while dancing, to place a handkerchief in their armpit and to flourish it later under the nose of the girl they admired in order to excite her sexually. Considered coldly, this seems to be a strange practice, but within the context of the general excitement of a social event such as a village festival it seems less unpleasant. We shall see in the next chapter that smells have a particular role to play in social gatherings. Returning to the exciting quality of underarm odor, it is well known that the duke of Anjou, later King Henri III of France, seized the discarded and sweaty chemise of his love, Marie de Clève, and drank in its odor with ecstatic delight.

An Expensive Enigma

The perfume industry today is worth thousands of millions of dollars annually in the Western world alone. Worldwide, it is worth an inestimable amount. Yet humans regard themselves as having poor noses. An expensive enigma, indeed! As we saw earlier, humans equate natural human odors with uncleanliness. Paradoxically, other odors are used as purifiers. It is virtually impossible nowadays to buy soap or a detergent or a floor polish that does not contain a "purifying" odor. Bacteriologists have had the greatest difficulty in dissuading surgeons from estimating the potency of a disinfectant by the strength of its smell, and every household disinfectant we can buy will proudly proclaim of what it smells.

Strong odors have been used since the earliest times to purge demons and cure diseases. If a treatment was to work, it had to smell. Odors, similarly, were thought to be able to protect people from illness when the Black Death swept Europe in the seventeenth century. Physicians held hollow sticks to their noses through which the odors of sandalwood and thyme could suffuse. And a London Bill of Mortality for 1635 gives precise instructions for the preparation of nosegays, which were supposed to protect their carriers from the scourge. "Take a

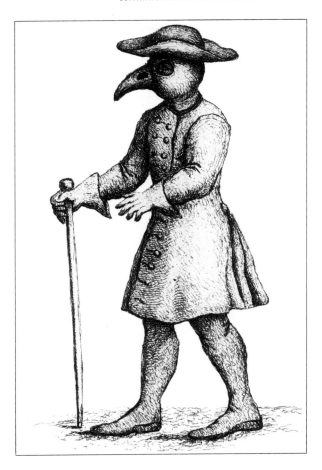

white sponge soaked in herb of grace water, which water is thus made: Take a quart of vinegar, half a pint of rose water, put in a handful of rice, and half a handful of wormwood, and boil it to a pint; then take and dip the sponge in it when it is cold, and hold it to your nose when you go abroad: and this is a good preservative." Alternatively, "Take of the best cedarwood, and grate a small wooden box full, and let the lid be full of holes and smell to it."

As we know from the contemporary children's nursery rhyme:

> Ring-a-ring-of-roses, a pocketful of posies,
> Atishoo, atishoo, we all fall down!

such scented trivia provided no protection at all, and the Black Death took whomsoever it wished. But it is fascinating to us now, with the benefit of modern knowledge, to realize that those who carried nosègays did so to satisfy one of the deepest longings in the human psyche.

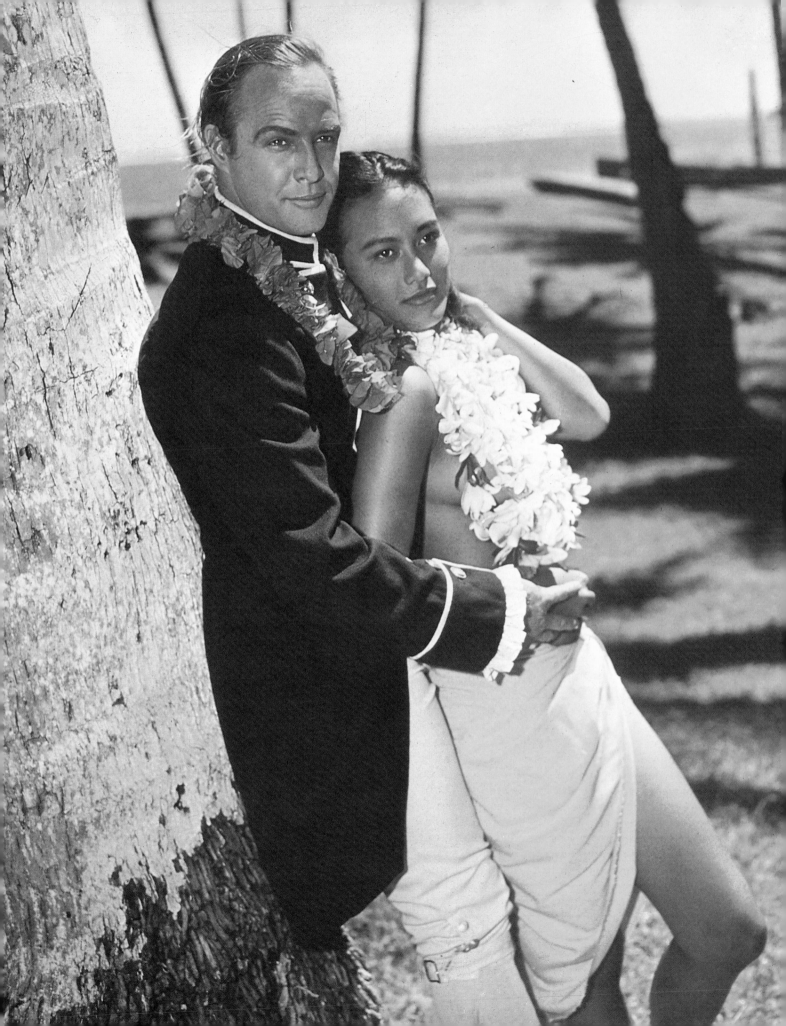

Chapter 9

Scent and Society

The greatest single difference between humans and animals is that humans can communicate abstract concepts to one another. The more highly civilized we are, the more we can afford to indulge in the luxuries of thought and social activity. Human social evolution has been astonishingly rapid — the Stone Age was only about 20,000 years ago. Borne along by the surging tide of civilization, man's ambivalent relationship with scent and smells found a fertile seedbed in his newly developing social activities and customs. And do not forget that the gregarious way of life is a human trait only recently acquired.

There are few peoples on the earth who have no religion at all. A deity has played a substantial role in human social evolution everywhere. Some religions may be thought of as brutal, demanding sacrifices of babies or old people, while others may be more comforting; but all probably help to keep human populations in harmony with the natural world. Even the most cursory glance over religions reveals a striking fact — in all of them odor plays an important part.

Some theologians have tried to analyze the role of scent in divine worship in terms of symbolism. For example, four of the ingredients of fragrant oil, identified by Moses prior to the flight from Egypt, were supposed to represent the four elements of land, water, fire and air. As we shall see, such analyses are unnecessary. A far simpler explanation is that man offers to the deity whatever he himself finds pleasing and, as we have already seen, he draws much of .his deepest emotional stimulation with every breath he breathes.

The Incense Cult

The scents and fragrances used in religious services are known collectively as incense, although the methods of preparation and burning differ markedly from one religion to the next. The earliest records of man's use of incense go back about six to seven

A scented garland of flowers, known as a lei, is a token of welcome or farewell in Hawaii. Given with a kiss, leis are living symbols of hospitality and friendship, a charming use of nature's perfumes. A visitor leaving Hawaii must toss the lei onto the water; if it floats to shore, the traveler will one day return to the Islands. Leis are made of scented flowers, often carnations, frangipane, jasmine, plumeria or orchids. Leis are also used as welcoming gifts in Tahiti, and in this image from Mutiny on the Bounty, *Marlon Brando (alias Fletcher Christian) is suitably adorned.*

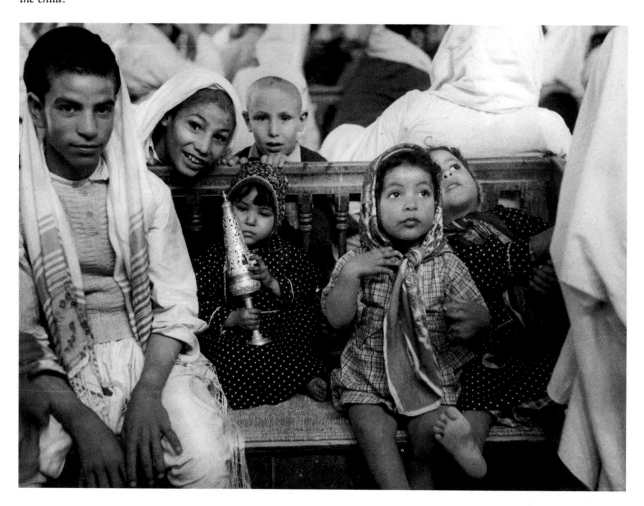

thousand years, to the Buddhists of China. All we know of the practices of those days is that various parts of plants were burned when all were gathered for worship. But we do know that the cult spread from the Chinese to the Indo-European races and received embellishment from the Hindus.

To obtain incense, the Hindus searched widely and established a trading route to and from the incense lands of Punt (now thought to be Somalia) in Africa. Here they sought frankincense, onycha, myrrh and aloes. Cassia was obtained from the East, even from China itself. The greatest contribution made by the Hindus was in the introduction of sandalwood to incense, and the delicate flowers of jasmine and spikenard.

From the Hindus, the cult spread westward and was adopted by the Egyptians. The first written record of the Egyptian use of incense in religious festivals dates from 3600 B.C., and the practice spread rapidly. By 3000 B.C., the office of "Chief of the House of Incense" existed, and it was the holder's duty to keep track of the supply and demand of incense. At the height of Egyptian power and influence — about 1500 B.C. — expeditions to the incense lands were undertaken on a truly vast scale. Men and donkeys trailed across the desert for months on end, seeking the gums and resins of the sacred incense-trees.

The main incense-tree is *Boswellia sacra*, and in the grandest expeditions whole trunks were loaded onto ships for transportation back to Alexandria. The incense-trees were guarded by austere, authoritarian families, who lived somber lives for fear of polluting the sacred resins. Shortly

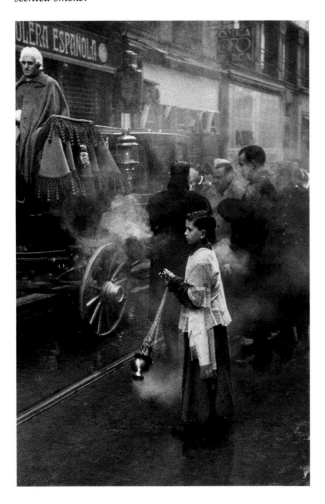

The young boy in the center of this Cartier-Bresson picture of a Madrid funeral holds a censer containing incense sprinkled on hot coals. He swings the censer to disperse the scented smoke.

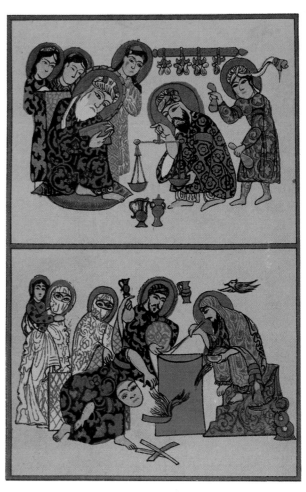

In this twelfth century manuscript, an Arab perfumer is shown making and selling his wares. The Arabs had long been makers of perfume and, as early as the thirteenth century, used distillation methods.

before resin was collected, they forsook all pleasures, hiding themselves away in a religious fervor. Rumors abounded that the trees were protected by a huge bat, which was said to tear out the eyes of anyone attempting to steal incense.

Cinnamon, which also grew in the land of Punt, was said to be the ground-up nest of the phoenix — a bird of profound mythological significance. Frankincense was thought to be the blood of an animate and divine plant. (This recalls the Islamic belief that, as Muhammad ascended to Heaven, he shed a tear upon the ground; from that spot a rose sprang up. To the Muslims, rose water, or water in which attar of roses — the essential rose oil — is dissolved, is symbolic of the prophet's tears.)

The Egyptians never strayed far from the odor of incense. Huge tributes of incense, fragrant oils and

spices were demanded from conquered peoples. During the annual feast of Baal, 1,000 talents (about 59 tons) of incense were burned on his great altar. In the three decades of his rule, King Rameses III reputedly reduced to ashes almost two million "pieces" of incense. It was the Egyptian habit to compound small cubes from ground-up incense, honey and the herb *Leptadenia pyrotechnica*. This herb contains nitric acid, which burns readily, helping the smoke to spiral upward. The cubes of incense were quite small — smaller than a gaming die — but nonetheless two million of them is a colossal quantity. As if to emphasize the social importance of odor, incense was burned only by kings and never by priests or ordinary mortals.

The Egyptians strongly believed that the gods exuded and exhaled sweet odors, and that security

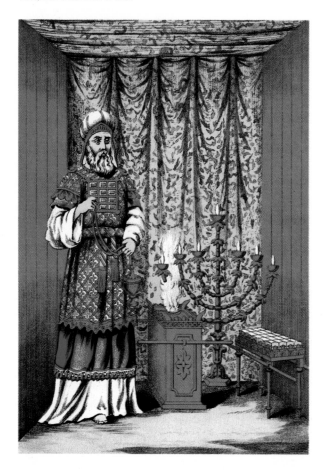

A Jewish high priest stands beside the altar of incense, the seven-branched candlestick and the table of showbread. The incense altar is thought to have been introduced between 300 and 2 B.C.

spiritual body made up of several components, whose eternal preservation was possible only if they were supported by the odor of incense. So, following death, incense was inserted into the body, and gums and resins were used to embalm it. Before being sealed in a sarcophagus, jars and pots of incense were placed beside the mummy as sustenance for the spiritual body. One tightly sealed pot, discovered in 1922 in the tomb of Tutankhamen, was analyzed and found to contain spikenard held in a neutral animal fat. Its potency was said to be high.

God's Instructions to Moses

As he led the Hebrews to the Holy Land, Moses was directed by God: "Take thou also unto thee these the principal spices, of pure myrrh five hundred shekels, and of sweet cinnamon half so much, even two hundred and fifty shekels, and of sweet calamus two hundred and fifty shekels. And of cassia five hundred shekels, after the shekel of the sanctuary, and of olive oil an hin. And thou shalt make of it an oil of holy anointment, an ointment compound after the art of the apothecary: it shall be an holy anointing oil." (Exodus 30: 23–5)

The instructions to Moses went farther, for he was to prepare a special perfume for use in the tabernacle: "And the Lord said unto Moses, take unto thee sweet spices, stacte and onycha and galbanum; these sweet spices with pure frankincense of each shall there be a like weight. And thou shalt make it a perfume, a confection after the art of the apothecary, tempered together, pure and holy. And thou shalt beat some of it very small and put it before the testimony in the tabernacle of the congregation, where I will meet with thee: it shall be unto you most holy." (Exodus 30: 34–6)

Before Solomon's temple was built in the ninth century B.C., the Hebrews worshipped on high places and humbled themselves before God by the interwoven rites of ceremonial prostitution and self-mutilation; prior to the writings of Jeremiah (628–586 B.C.) the Hebrews were not known to use incense in the way it is used at present. By the time of the diaspora, however, the Jews had a good grasp of incense rites, presumably learned from Egyptians and wandering traders from the Orient. Sometime between 300 B.C. and 2 B.C. a special

in the afterlife could be assured if heavenly odors could enter the human body. Isis was said to impart her wonderful odor to the dead, and Osiris could transfer his odor to those whom he loved. We know that, immediately after death, a rite called "The Chapter of the Opening of the Mouth" was performed to assure the deceased's passage to heaven. A papyrus from the time tells us that a priest made this incantation: "The perfume of Arabia has been brought to thee, to make perfect thy smell through the scent of the God. Here are brought to thee liquids which are come from Ra, to make perfect thy smell in the Hall of Judgement. O, sweet-smelling souls of the Great God, thou dost contain such a sweet odor that thy face shall neither change nor perish."

It is not surprising, then, that the Egyptians took to embalming the dead in incense resins. They believed that, besides his earthly body, man had a

Floral offerings and perfumed cloths were used in the mummification rituals of ancient Egypt. Sweet smells were thought to appease the gods and help the body's passage into heaven.

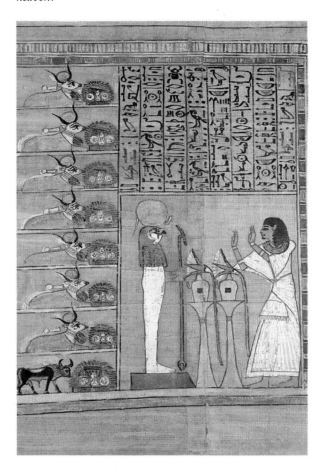

incense altar was introduced, and an elegant construction of cedarwood and gold it was.

If Homer's *Illiad* is to be believed, perfumes played no part in the savage and bestial society of the early days of the Greek Empire. But the expansion of the empire in 700–600 B.C. brought the Greeks into contact with the Egyptians, and in just the same way in which they had learned of incense from traders from the East, so the Greeks acquired their knowledge from the Egyptians. Writing in the fifth century B.C., Euripides refers to Syria as the source of frankincense and other fragrant substances.

Incense in the Classical World
In the second century B.C., Theophrastus, who wrote extensively about plants, was considering the significance of smells quite deeply. According to Aristophanes, the Greeks used incense in powdered form, sprinkled onto glowing charcoal,

which suggests that the early Christians acquired their knowledge from the Greeks rather than from the Egyptians, who persisted with blocks of self-burning incense.

As the Greek Empire expanded, odors were used excessively, and no opportunity was wasted, either public or private, to anoint guests with scented oils or to burn incense. The guests of the Greek king of Syria, Antiochus Epiphanes, were greeted by two hundred girls, who sprayed and sprinkled rose water, and a similar number of boys, who carried braziers containing myrrh, frankincense, sandalwood and other aromatic resins.

A Homage to Gods and Nobles
Farther west, the youthful Roman Empire had embarked upon an expansionist policy, and, by the last century before Christ's birth, had incorporated many uses of incense into its rites. The naturalist, Pliny the Elder (A.D. *c.*23–79), tells us that the fragrance of cedar and other woods was well known.

Incense was burned in temples as a specific homage to the gods, but, significantly, it was more heavily used on grand state occasions. When a general returned triumphant to Rome after a successful and distant campaign, the route into the city was lined with censer (incense) bearers, and the general floated on a veritable cloud of incense. Vast quantities of incense were used on these occasions, but it was only a fraction of what had been used daily throughout the Greek Empire.

When the Romans took over the regions of Magna Graecia in southern Italy after the fall of Antioch, they were disgusted by what they saw as a perfumed, feminized society. In 188 B.C. an edict was issued from Rome forbidding the use of incense on a large scale, but the warning was soon forgotten. Two centuries later, at the funeral of Nero's wife Poppaea, many tons of incense were used. The supply of the precious ingredients from Arabia was not inexhaustible, and, as the cost rose, the Roman Treasury shuddered. Some historians believe that the vast cost of incense was a major contributory factor in the chronic economic problems that accompanied, and perhaps even brought about, the collapse of the Empire.

Undoubtedly the heavy use made of incense by the Jews at the time of Christ's betrayal was the

151

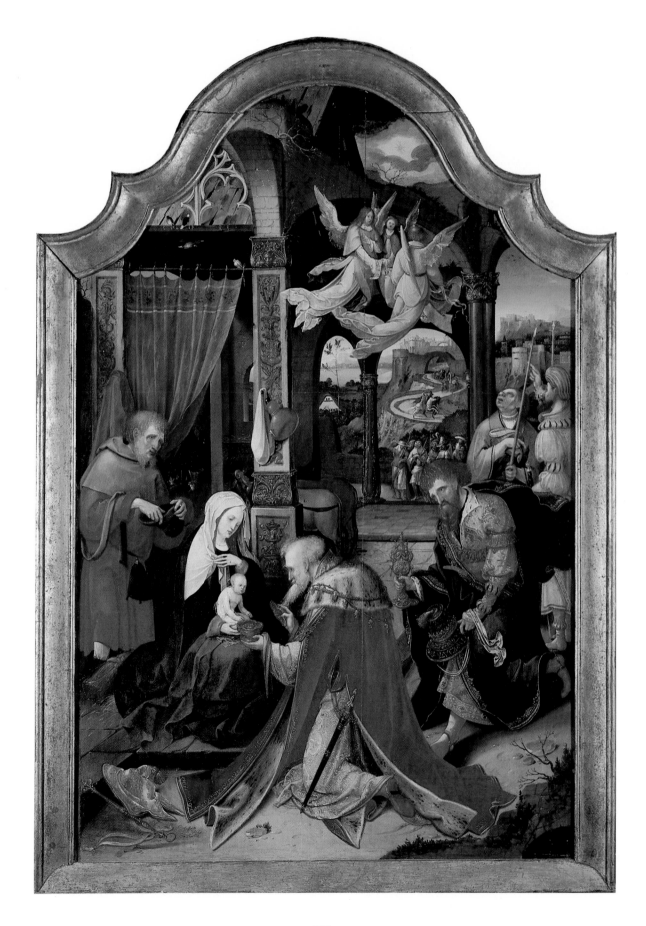

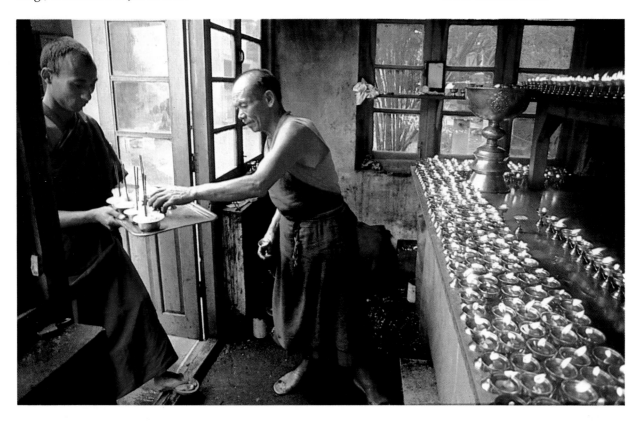

reason for the complete rejection of the practice during the first few centuries of Christianity. An extremely perceptive Syrian Christian, Arnobius, asked a number of questions about the use of incense that are of particular significance and are as penetrating today as when they were first formulated. Querying whether the gods needed smoke to placate them, he wrote: ''What is this sign of respect which comes from the smell of gum of a tree burning in a fire? Does this, do you suppose, give honour to the heavenly magnates? Or if their displeasure has been aroused at any time, is it really soothed and dissipated by incense smoke? But if it is smoke that the gods want, why do you not offer them any sort of smoke? Or must it only be incense? If you answer that incense has a nice smell while other substances have not, tell me if the gods have nostrils, and can they smell with them? But if the gods are incorporeal, odours and perfumes can have no effect at all on them, since corporeal substances cannot affect incorporeal beings.''

The same theme was taken up by St. Basil the

Great in the middle of the fourth century. He says: ''Incense is now an abomination unto the Lord. For truly it is an execrable thing to think that God values the pleasures of the sense of smell, and not to understand that the hallowing of the body, effected by the sobriety of the soul, is the incense unto the Lord. Corporeal incense that affects the nostrils and moves the senses is by a necessary consequence regarded as an abomination to a Being that is incorporeal.''

The sharp logic underlying Arnobius' and St. Basil's writings confirms what we already know: men offer incense because they themselves gain inspiration from it. This is the sole motivation for its appearance. Notice that St. Basil knew that the smell of incense was capable of moving the senses — by this he was inferring that conscious control of human emotion was threatened by the odor. In spite of these and other protests against incense, by the fourth or fifth century A.D. incense rites had crept into the Christian religion, and all opposition fell away. In the Catholic church today, incense

People surround a steaming caldron of incense during a ritual in the Ueno Park Temple in Tokyo. Tradition says that placing incense on the head brings cleverness, on the face, beauty and on the body, health.

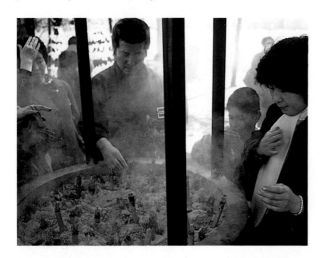

rites have become almost as complex as they were in the Egyptian temple of Herod, in the eighteenth century B.C.

A Scourge on Evil

It is not just in the world's great religions that incense plays a role. In every form of pagan ceremony, incense is used to purify and placate. In a number of areas, it is believed that departed spirits of the dead can be summoned by a medium, who first prepares him- or herself by deeply inhaling the fumes of incense. In Kashmir, the incense is the smoke of cedarwood; farther east, the fortune teller may drink in the heavy odor of sandalwood.

In all instances of mediums making contact with the dead, we find that incense fulfills two functions. First, it allows the medium's own spirit to take a temporary vacation, thereby permitting the spirit of the dead person to enter a vacant body that has a voice box and a tongue. And second, it serves to protect the medium by warding off evil spirits. (Is this not reminiscent of the strong odor of antiseptics?) In the Kei Islands, near New Guinea, evil spirits form a mighty host, inhabiting every tree, cave and pile of stones. As they can easily be offended, and as their wrath is tremendous, the antidote is to burn some scrapings from a buffalo's horn or, in earlier times, some hair from a Papuan slave, for the foul pungent proteinaceous smell will feed the evil spirits and divert their attention from fearful people.

These tribal practices remind us of what we know

the Egyptians believed: that evil was associated with bad odor, while goodness was identified by sweet odor. Sweet odors form one of the characteristics of Hindu and Buddhist paradises: when divine beings descend to malodorous hell, they change the foul odor to a sweet one by vanquishing evil. In ancient Canton, incense was used to guard against specific demons — one particular mixture was even said to protect against poverty. Because evil flees before its sweet odor, incense is a most important constituent of the amulet box of Tibet, without which no person would dare to undertake a hazardous journey.

Among various African tribes, it is not uncommon for a rank and fetid-smelling billy goat to be tied to the bed of a demented person. Then, a few hours later, the medicine man brings some sweet-smelling herbs into the afflicted person's hut, which scares the demon, causing it to seek refuge in the goat, for the rancid-smelling beast now appears as a haven to the evil spirit. After killing the poor goat, and, of course, the demon within it, the afflicted person is declared clean.

A vibrant and clear theme runs through all these anecdotes. Incense is associated with a state of mind which humans find comforting and thus, when in its presence, there is no room for evil, which causes spiritual and, in many cultures, physical discomfort. So what precisely is it about incense that makes it so powerful? Remember that fifteen hundred years ago Arnobius asked this question, and St. Basil recognized that its odor could deeply affect the mind.

Incense and the Human Mind

A striking feature of all incense recipes is that just a handful of ingredients has been included, irrespective of where in the world the incense is used. As was mentioned earlier, the Hindus did add certain other substances to the basic ingredients of incense, but over the centuries such additions have been remarkably few. Most ingredients are gums and resins from various plants, though powdered wood and roots also occur.

Resins are complex chemicals, having a structure resembling that of the animal steroids — the group of compounds which, we saw earlier, are found in sex hormones and in animal, and perhaps

Name	Alternative names	Substance	Source
Styrax	Storax, stacte	Resin	*Styrax officialis, Liquidambar orientalis*; Middle East, India
Onycha	Incense nail, sea clove	Keratinized protein	Opercula of snail, *Unguis odoratus*; Red Sea
Galbanum	Asafoetida, Heart resin	Resin	*Ferula galbanifula, F. rhinocaulis*; Middle East
Frankincense	Olibanum	Resin	*Boswellia sacra, B. carteri*; Southeast Arabia
Myrrh	Balsam, balm, bdellium	Resin	*Commiphora myrrha, C. molmo*; Middle East to Pakistan
Sweet cinnamon	Ceylonese cinnamon	Bark	*Cinnamomum zeylanicum*; Sri Lanka, India
Cassia	Chinese cinnamon	Bark	*Cinnamomum cassia*; S. China
Sweet cane	Calmus	Rhizome	*Acorus calamus*; Central Asia
Gum benzoin	Benzoin	Gum	*Styrax benzoin*; India, Far East
Aloes	Eaglewood, Lign-aloe	Wood	*Aquilaria agallochum*; Arabia, Middle East, India
Tragacanth		Resin	*Astragalus gummifer*; Middle East
Spikenard	Nard	Stem	*Nardostacys jatamansi*; Himalayas
Ladanum	Laudanum	Resin	*Cistus ladaniferus*; Middle East
Cedar		Wood	*Juniperus virginiana*; worldwide
Sandal	White sandal	Wood	*Santalum album*; India
Costus		Root	*Auklandia costus*; Middle East
Saffron		Pollen	*Crocus sativus*; Iran, Pakistan
Mace		Seedcoat of nutmeg	*Myristica fragrans*; East Indies
Jasmine		Flowers	

also human, pheromones. Is it possible that the secret of the power of incense is that it is a pheromone mimic? Is this why men everywhere praise the deity with just those specific materials and none other? Is this why they deeply influence the working of the human mind in the way St. Basil feared? There is some evidence that this may be so.

The Dutch psychiatrist Professor J. Kloek asked a large group of students from the University of Utrecht to sniff a series of steroids and then to record their impressions according to a number of

The main ingredients of incense, the plants from which they are obtained and the areas from which they come are shown in the table. The first eight of these ingredients were indicated to Moses prior to the Exodus. Galbanum, according to Pliny, was incorporated into incense, not for its strong, pungent odor, but to make sweet spices retain their fragrance longer.

headings, for example, the odor is most like meat, dead leaves, sweat etc. He was interested to find that a consistently high proportion of students thought the steroids smelled of "sandalwood" — one of his response categories. Drawing attention to this, Kloek states: "Very interesting is the woody odor (cedarwood, sandalwood) of some steroids, in connection with the fact that the delicate scents of some trees seem to be important in many religious cults. In our investigation, it happened several times that a smell was called "like incense," which, very probably, may be interpreted as "like cedar- or sandalwood," as powdered cedarwood is used for incense."

In a further, perhaps more subjective, test, the Austrian perfumer Dr. Paul Jellinek took a number of incense ingredients and described them in terms of human odor. Styrax, he said, smelled like the skin of dark-haired people; frankincense recalled the sebum of dark- and red-haired subjects. The sebum of blond people smelled like myrrh, while head hair of all people smelled like ladanum. Finally, he noted that costus smelled like the axillary organ secretion of dark-haired subjects.

Such a test cannot be free from the bias caused by ordinary human experience, but nevertheless, as a trained perfumer, Jellinek is well qualified to point out odor similarities. In his writings, he frequently refers to the "erotic" enhancement of perfumes by the mixing of various ingredients with floral eaux-de-cologne. Interestingly, he notes a strong enhancement of the erotic nature of floral perfumes when incense ingredients are added. Again, such an assessment cannot be free from his personal bias, but it is certainly an assessment worthy of further consideration.

Weaving all these strands of evidence and observation together, we can begin to formulate a hypothesis explaining why a handful of natural plant products should have played such a dominant role in human social behavior through the ages. We have already seen that humans no longer respond to sexual odors in the way their ancestors did, and other mammals still do.

Community living, such that large prey could be tackled, meant that the sense of smell became repressed, to ensure that families remained as families and that females kept their sexual favors for their recognized mates alone. Masking of their sexual odors, which broadcast ovulation and the heat, was enhanced by the earliest of all perfumes — fruit and leaf juices. Much later, when natural selection had firmly fitted the lid of smell repression onto the human psyche, the memory traces of the past could be tugged a little by the use of animal sex-attractant products in perfumes.

Incense serves exactly the same function. Its ingredients smell not unlike steroids and serve to focus the mind on the events going on all around. St. Basil was right — the mind *is* deeply stirred by incense — but it is doubtful if he knew in which area of human biology the disturbance lay. The use of incense is an extremely subtle and sublime form of the use of sex in advertising the social nature of events.

Minds are sharpened and altered in the presence of incense, and, in this state, they attain a level of comfort and of sensual well-being in which the future can be faced. This is only a hypothesis, but it fits the facts. Much more work needs to be done by chemists and physiologists before we can be sure that incense is truly a pheromone mimic.

Why no Odor Culture?

In one final respect, the sense of smell is quite different from its cousins of sight and hearing, and is even different from its twin — taste. Human culture all over the world, and in myriad ways, has elaborated the hedonic side of the senses. Great artists paint magnificent pictures, and composers write reams of music, which fill the concert hall to bursting point with a glorious burgeoning of sound. Cordon bleu chefs create special dishes, and vintners fine wines, to titillate the sense of taste. Yet we have no odor culture. Of course, there are great creators of fine perfumes, but, as we saw earlier, these are designed for close relations, and their names suggest intimacy. Just compare the name of the scent, *"Intimate"* with that of the symphony, *"Eroica."*

Odor culture, such as it is, is only expressed relatively privately. Will the time ever come when huge fans at railroad stations and airports will waft perfumes down the concourses, just as today loudspeakers produce "canned" music? Probably not. As far as is known, only once in the history of

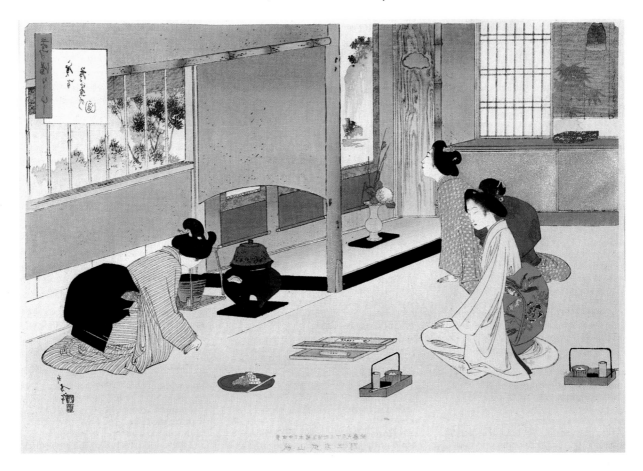

mankind has an odor art evolved, but already its popularity has declined.

It was performed in Japan, often in tea houses and under the direction of the tea masters. Participants prepared for the event a full day before by not smoking, drinking neither saki nor tea, eating no aromatic foods and using no perfume. After bathing, they dressed in clean kimonos and went to the tea house. There they shed their outer garments, which might have become contaminated with street odors.

When all were assembled, the tea master produced a censer containing a mixture of four ingredients, three of which had been passed around immediately prior to the test. The guests used their powers of recall to name the fourth ingredient and put forward their assessments to the master by way of a complicated series of tablets and slips of paper. At the end of each ceremony, a prize was awarded to the participant making the highest number of correct determinations. In many respects, this form of art is similar to the type of theatrical performance favored by the Ancient Greeks, in which the audience actively participated and so left the performance spiritually enriched.

It is a matter of some shame that the art of the tea ceremony was castigated by Europeans, who considered it trivial and the product of social decadence: but this was probably because the sense of smell plays no part in Western culture, other than in churches. There is no simple reason to explain why odor culture has not been developed elsewhere, but it is probably something to do with our enigmatic attitude to smell. We do not wish to be reminded of our animal origins, and we are afraid of what smells may teach us about ourselves. Smell remains the last great taboo, about which "nice" people remain silent.

Glossary

acoustic energy the energy of sound waves that causes the eardrum to vibrate.

amplitude the breadth of vibration of a wave — the vertical distance from peak to trough.

amygdala a nucleus of nerve cells at the base of each cerebral hemisphere, adjacent to the hypothalamus. An important relay station for olfactory and gustatory impulses.

androstenes a family of steroids responsible for the odor emanating from the axillary glands in the armpit.

ano-genital region the part of the body including the anus and genitals.

anosmia complete loss of the sense of smell.

apical pore the entrance to a taste bud.

apocrine gland a skin gland found particularly in the hairy parts of the body and responsible for producing a fatty secretion containing odorous substances.

audiogram a graph of the minimum sound levels required to detect a sound at various frequencies and used by audiologists to describe the competence of an ear.

audiologist an investigator of normal and abnormal hearing.

auditory cortex the part of the cerebral cortex in which sounds are perceived and interpreted.

axilla the armpit, the skin of which is equipped with abundant apocrine and sweat glands.

axon the long fiber of a nerve cell, stretching from the nerve cell body and making a synaptic contact with another nerve or with a muscle.

basal cells small, young cells in the olfactory membrane and taste bud.

basilar membrane the all-important membrane in the cochlea which responds to sounds of different frequencies by exhibiting vibration patterns called traveling waves.

Bel a unit describing a tenfold increase in sound intensity.

bony labyrinth the bony cavity in which the cochlea and semicircular canals lie.

carotenoids a ubiquitous family of chemical pigments responsible for many of the reds, yellows and oranges in nature.

cerebellum the part of the brain coordinating the nervous impulses which control the muscles and joints involved in movement, balance and posture.

cerebral cortex the thin layer of gray matter covering both cerebral hemispheres in which all the higher functions of brain activity are carried out.

ceruminous glands glands in the ear canal or auditory meatus which produce wax or cerumen.

chemoreception the reception of chemical stimuli by the nose and by the taste buds.

chorda tympani a branch of the facial nerve (cranial nerve) mainly concerned with relaying information to the brain about salt and sweet chemoreception.

cilia microscopical hairlike processes of many cell types. Cilia may be motile or be involved in a cell's responsiveness to stimuli.

cochlea the snail-shaped part of the inner ear in which the organ of hearing is housed.

cochlear duct see scala media.

concha one of the scroll-like bony flaps on the side of each nostril. Also the conical hole leading from the external ear to the ear canal.

conductive hearing loss the loss of hearing resulting from the decreased mobility of the ossicles situated in the middle ear.

cranial nerve one of the twelve pairs of nerves leaving the underside of the brain and leading to various parts of the body.

cribriform plate a small waferthin patch of the ethmoid bone. Through its sievelike structure the receptor cells in the olfactory membranes below it make nervous connections with the olfactory bulbs above.

cytoplasm the parts of a cell outside the nucleus.

decibel (dB) a unit measurement of the intensity or pressure level of a sound. One tenth of a Bel.

distillation the process of extracting essential oils from their organic source.

echolocation the accurate method of pinpointing objects achieved by emitting very high frequency sound waves and then receiving their echoes.

ectoderm the outer of the three basic layers of embryological tissue, from which the nervous system, sense organs, skin, hair, teeth and nails develop.

electron microscopy microscopy using electron beams which enable much higher magnifications to be usefully achieved than are possible with optical microscopes.

electrophysiology the study of the electrical phenomena in cells such as nerves and muscles in order to discover their operation and function.

endolymph the fluid in the scala media.

enfleurage the process used by the Arabs and Persians of the Middle Ages to extract plant odors for use in perfumes.

entorhinal cortex an olfactory center of a high order located in the hippocampal region of the brain.

epiglottis a small leaf-shaped cartilage attached to the thyroid cartilage in the larynx which moves up and down to prevent food and drink from entering the trachea.

epithelium a surface layer of cells on most internal and external systems of the body.

esophagus the gullet: a tube which in man is about ten inches long and extends from the pharynx to the stomach.

essential oil the concentrated extract of a plant odor dissolved in alcohol.

estrus the cycle of events in the female reproductive organs of mammals. To be "in estrus" is to be "in heat".

Eustachian tube the canal joining the middle ear cavity to the nasopharynx.

filiform papillae the most numerous of the various papillae of the tongue. They are not involved in the perception of taste but rather have an abrasive function.

foliate papillae leaflike papillae found roughly in the middle of each side of the tongue.

frequency the number of sound waves passing a particular point in one second. Measured in cycles per second or in Hertz (Hz).

frenulum linguae a mucous membrane fold under the tongue which holds the tongue to the floor of the mouth.

fungiform papillae tiny mushroom-like papillae scattered over the surface of the tongue.

ganglion clusters of nerve cell bodies found outside the brain and spinal cord.

genio-glossus an extrinsic muscle found on each side of the tongue.

glomeruli the sites in the olfactory bulb where primary neurones from the receptor cells make synapses with tufted cells and with secondary olfactory neurones.

glosso-pharyngeal nerve   the IXth cranial nerve which relays taste information from the rear third of the tongue and from the pharynx to the brain.
glossal   pertaining to the tongue.
glycoprotein   a protein with sugar molecules bound to it.
gustation   the sense of taste.

harmonic   a sound frequency which is an exact multiple of a fundamental frequency.
Hertz (Hz)   a measure of frequency where one Hertz is one cycle per second.
hyoid bone   a U-shaped bone in the throat.
hyo-glossus   an extrinsic muscle found on each side of the tongue.
hypothalamus   a small but vital area located beneath the thalamus and on the floor of the brain's third ventricle. One of its many roles is to relay information about chemoreception to the brain's higher centers.

incus   the "anvil" bone of the middle ear.
intensity   the loudness, or pressure level, of a sound measured in decibels.
ion   a positively or negatively charged atom, such as the cation Na$^+$ and the anion Cl$^-$.
ionic exchange   the transport of ions across the membrane of a nerve or receptor cell before and after the passage of an evoked action potential.

kilohertz (kHz)   a frequency of 1000 cycles per second.

labyrinth   the maze of bony and membranous passages of the inner ear.
larynx   the voice box, lying below the root of the tongue, above the trachea and in front of the lowest part of the pharynx.
limbic system   one of the "oldest" parts of the brain which forms a ring-like base to the cerebral hemispheres and functions on the level of emotional and sexual behavior.
loudness discomfort level   the level of intensity, on average about 100 decibels, at which the sensation of sound causes discomfort.
lymphoid nodules   the clusters of lingual tonsils at the back of the tongue, which trap and kill bacteria.

malleus   the "hammer" bone of the middle ear.
median furrow   the visible groove down the middle of the tongue.

median septum   the fibrous division of the two halves of the tongue lying below the median furrow.
medulla   the lowest part of the brain stem where the spinal cord ends and the brain begins.
membranous labyrinth   the system of sacs and spaces within the bony labyrinth of the inner ear which houses the receptor cells of the cochlear and vestibular systems and which contains endolymph.
microtubules   submicroscopic tubular organelles within the cytoplasm of cells.
microvilli   small fingerlike projections at the surfaces of cells.
midbrain   the uppermost part of the brain stem lying immediately below the cerebral hemispheres.
mitosis   the division of a cell nucleus into two identical daughter nuclei — usually followed by cell division.
molarity   the concentration of a particular substance where a molarity of one is expressed as the molecular weight in grams dissolved in a liter of water.
molecule   the smallest mass of any substance which still retains the properties of that substance.
monosaccharide   a simple sugar.
mucous membrane   the lining of the nose and mouth which typically secretes mucus.
mucus   the viscous fluid secreted by mucous membranes.
myelin   the fatty sheath surrounding and insulating the axons of many nerve fibers, enabling nerve impulses to travel at high speeds.

nasopharynx   the top part of the pharynx extending from the back of the nose to the level of the soft palate.
neurologist   a nerve specialist.
neurone   a nerve cell.
neurophysiologist   a specialist in the operation and function of nerves.

odor fatigue   the adaptation of the nose to a particular odor so that, after a while, the odor is not perceived.
olfaction   the sense of smell.
olfactometry   the measurement of the olfactory sense.
olfactory bulb   the part of the brain, lying above the cribriform plate, which receives nerve fibers from the olfactory membrane.
olfactory clefts   two narrow cavities lying each side of the nasal septum at the very top of the nose, in which the olfactory membranes lie.

olfactory hairs   the microscopic strands, or cilia, which emerge from the receptor cells of the olfactory membrane and are directly stimulated by molecules of odor.
olfactory imprinting   the deep impression made by a mother's odor on her newborn, suckling child.
olfactory lobes   the olfactory bulbs.
olfactory membrane   a patch of yellow-gray tissue, situated high in the olfactory cleft, containing millions of receptor cells and even more olfactory hairs.
olfactory mucosa   the olfactory membrane.
olfactory neurone   one of the nerve fibers leading from the receptors in the olfactory membrane to the olfactory bulb and from there to the olfactory centers in the brain.
organ of Corti   the organ of hearing in the cochlea of the ear.
ossicles   the three tiny bones of the middle ear.
otitis media   a bacterial infection in which the lining of the middle ear swells, so impairing the action of the ossicles.
otoliths   the tiny calcareous crystals found in the vestibular apparatus of the inner ear. They move about in the endolymph and trigger receptor cells in response to gravity and linear movements of the head.
otologist   a physician specializing in disorders of the ear.
otosclerosis   a serious condition in which new bone grows over the stapes bone of the middle ear and impairs its movement, causing partial or total deafness.
oval window   the membranous partition between the stapes bone and the scala vestibuli of the cochlea.

palatine   pertaining to the palate
palato-glossals   a pair of extrinsic muscles of the tongue. Together they lift the sides of the tongue.
papillae   the tiny elevations that cover the upper surface of the tongue. There are four types — filiform, fungiform, foliate and vallate — of which the last three contain taste buds.
perilymph   the fluid filling the scala vestibuli and the scala tympani.
period   the repeat duration of a sound wave in time.
pharynx   the throat.
pheromone   a chemical, which signals from one individual to another an internal physiological change or a change in behavior.

phon a measure of subjective loudness level.

phonemes the sounds of speech.

phospholipid a chemical combination of fatty acids and phosphate.

pinna the external ear.

pitch the mind's interpretation of the frequency of a sound.

pituitary organ the master gland of the endocrine system, whose hormones control the secretions of other endocrine glands and are, in turn, controlled by the hypothalamus.

psychophysics the study of the relationship between the psychological and physical aspects of a stimulus. The quantification of perception.

psychophysiology the study of the relationship between the psychological and physiological aspects of a response to a stimulus.

pulse labeling the experimental use of a short period of exposure to radioactive isotopes of atoms.

radioisotope the radioactive isotope of an atom. For example, tritium is a radioisotope of hydrogen.

rarefaction the thinning out of air molecules caused by the passage of a sound wave.

receptor cells cells specialized to respond to particular stimuli by initiating electrical responses.

Reissner's membrane the membrane dividing the scala vestibuli from the scala media in the inner ear.

respiratory mucosa a specialized mucous membrane that makes mucus and possesses many cilia which move the mucus back to the nasopharynx.

rhinologist a nose specialist.

Riechlust the pleasure young children under the age of five derive from their sense of smell.

round window a membranous partition at the bottom end of the scala tympani, which allows pressure in the perilymph to escape into the middle ear and from there into the Eustachian tube and nasopharynx.

scala media the cochlear duct containing the auditory hair cells.

scala tympani the descending space of the cochlea which is filled with perilymph; it begins at the apex of the cochlea and winds down to the round window.

scala vestibuli the ascending space of the cochlea which is filled with perilymph; it begins at the oval window and winds up to the apex of the cochlea.

sebaceous gland a skin gland which is associated with hair follicles and produces sebum.

sebum a fatty secretion containing cell debris from the sebaceous glands which conditions and waterproofs hair.

semicircular canals the three loops of the vestibular apparatus set at right angles to one another and responsible for sensing movements of the head in three dimensions.

sensorineural hearing loss loss of hearing due to damaged hair cells in the organ of Corti or damaged cochlear nerve fibers.

sine wave the sinuous up-and-down shape that describes the oscillation between two opposing states, such as the compression and rarefaction of air during the passage of a sound wave.

sinusoidal waveform a sine wave.

soft palate the muscular partition, shaped like an arch, which divides the mouth from the nasopharynx.

sound pressure level (SPL) the intensity of a sound.

stapedectomy the removal of the stapes bone and its replacement with a metal or plastic prosthesis.

stapedius muscle the muscle which attaches the stapes to the wall of the middle ear cavity and which contracts to immobilize the stapes.

stapes the "stirrup" bone of the middle ear.

stereochemistry the area of chemistry based on the various shapes and configurations of molecules.

steroid a family of chemicals occurring naturally in the body including the sex hormones, cholesterol and the corticosteroid hormones.

stylo-glossals a pair of extrinsic muscles of the tongue. Together these muscles pull the tongue backward and upward.

subcortical projections the nerve connections between an organ, such as the tongue, and evolutionarily ancient areas of the brain beneath the cerebral cortex, such as the medulla, pons, hypothalamus and amygdala.

synapse a region of close contact and communication between two nerve cells.

tastant molecule the molecule of a substance, such as sugar, that creates a taste sensation by stimulating the taste buds.

taste bud the microscopic clusters of sensory cells specifically responsible for gustatory chemoreception by the tongue.

tectorial membrane a gelatinous membrane in the organ of Corti to which the hairs of the outer hair cell receptors are attached.

temporary threshold shift the increase in loudness needed to hear normal sounds after the ear has been subjected to high noise levels.

tensor tympani muscle the muscle attached via a long ligament to the malleus. It contracts in response to very loud noises, pulling the arm of the malleus to increase tension in the eardrum.

thalamus the part of the brain situated below the cerebral hemispheres and above the midbrain. It is a major relay station in the passage of sensory information to the cerebral cortex.

tinnitus spontaneous and persistent ringing in the ears.

tone decay test a clinical test for damage to the cochlear nerve which measures how long it takes for the perception of a tone of constant intensity to decline.

traveling wave the complex pattern of vibrations set up in the basilar membrane in response to pressure changes in the cochlear fluid.

tympanum/tympanic membrane the eardrum.

uvula the visible cone-shaped projection suspended from the midpoint of the soft palate arch at the back of the mouth.

vallate papillae the largest of the papillae, numbering from seven to twelve on the human tongue and located in a V-shape toward the back of the tongue.

vestibular apparatus the part of the inner ear not concerned with hearing but with balance and orientation of the head.

vestibular labyrinth the system of spaces, loops and sacs in which the semicircular canals and other parts of the vestibular apparatus are situated.

wavelength the distance between two peaks of a wave, such as two adjacent areas of compression in a sound wave.

white noise noise which is made up of energy across a wide range of frequencies.

X-ray diffraction crystallography a method of determining the 3-D shape of molecules by studying the way in which a crystal of those molecules diffracts a beam of X-rays.

Illustration Credits

Introduction
6, Mary Evans Picture Library.

The Functioning of the Ear
8, Printed by permission of the Estate of Norman Rockwell, Copyright © 1948 Estate of Norman Rockwell. 10, (left) BBC Hulton Picture Library, (right) Zimberoff/Liason/ Frank Spooner Pictures. 11, *The Annunciation* by El Greco. Illescas, Toledo/Michael Holford. 12, (left) Mansell Collection, (right) Wellcome Institute Library, London. 13, Ann Ronan Picture Library. 14, *The Garden of Earthly Delights: Musical Hell* by Hieronymus Bosch. Prado, Madrid/Bridgeman Art Library. 15, **Michael Woods**. 16, Kim Taylor/ Bruce Coleman Limited. 17, Ann Ronan Picture Library. Foldout, (outside) Dr. G. Bredberg, South Hospital, Stockholm, Sweden, (inside) **Frank Kennard**. 18, Ann Ronan Picture Library. 19, Ann Ronan Picture Library. 20, (both) Jane Burton/Bruce Coleman Limited. 21, *States of Mind I* by Umberto Boccioni. Private Collection, New York/Scala. 22, **Norman Barber**. 23, (all) Ann Ronan Picture Library. 24, Bildarchiv Preussischer Kulturbesitz. 25, courtesy of HMV. 26, (left) Rick Smolan/Contact/Colorific, (right) Wil Blanche/Rex Features. 27, John Watney Photo Library. 28, **Mike Courtney**. 29, Wellcome Institute Library, London. 30, **Mike Courtney**. 31, UCLA School of Medicine/ Science Photo Library. 32, Sherman Hines/ Masterfile/Daily Telegraph Colour Library. 33, Mansell Collection.

Sound and Hearing
34, *The Scream* by Edvard Munch. National Gallery, Oslo/Bridgeman Art Library. 36, (top) **Michael Woods**, (bottom) BBC Hulton Picture Library. 37, **Michael Woods**. 38, **Michael Woods**. 39, Don Hunstein/Colorific. 40, Associated Press. 41, *Liszt on the Piano* by Josef Danhauser. Nationalgalerie Staatliche Museen Preussischer Kulturbesitz, Berlin. 42, (top) KRESGE Hearing Research Institute, University of Michigan Medical School; courtesy Professor Joseph E. Hawkins; SEM Robert E. Preston, (bottom) BBC Hulton Picture Library. 43, **Michael Woods**. 44, (top) **Michael Woods**, (bottom) Dr. Harold Edgerton, MIT/Science Photo Library. 46, Lee E. Battaglia/Colorific. 47, John Topham Picture Library. 48, (both) **Michael Woods**. 49, R. Creamer/Sygma/The John Hillelson Agency. 50, (left) Richard Bryant/ ARCAID, (right) John Topham Picture Library. 51, Gillian D. Sales.

The Imperfect Ear
52, *Beethoven* by Lucien Lévy-Dhurmer. Petit Palais/Bulloz. 54, (top) Adam Woolfitt/Susan Griggs Agency, (bottom, both) Ann Ronan Picture Library. 55, (top left) Gene Cox/ Science Photo Library, (top right) Dr. Tony Brain, Chelsea College of Science and Technology, London/Science Photo Library, (bottom right) Gene Cox/Science Photo Library. 56, *Story of a Widow III* by Pavel Nesleha/ Bridgeman Art Library. 57, P. J. Martin/Royal National Institute for the Deaf, London. 58, (left) John Watney Photo Library, (right) P. J.

Martin/Royal National Institute for the Deaf, London. 59, Thomas Hopker/The John Hillelson Agency. 60, (left) **Michael Woods**, (right) BBC Hulton Picture Library. 61, Ann Ronan Picture Library. 62, *A Concert* by Carmontelle. Musée Condé, Chantilly/Bulloz. 63, (top) British Museum/Michael Holford, (bottom) Erich Lessing/Magnum/The John Hillelson Agency.

The Versatile Tongue
64, Anwar Hussein. 66, (left) Adrian Davies/ Bruce Coleman Limited, (right) Martin Dohrn/Science Photo Library. 67, **Mike Courtney**. 68, *Mick Jagger* (1975) by Andy Warhol © DACS 1984. 69, Ronald Sheridan Photo Library. 70, Ronald Sheridan Photo Library. 71, Victoria and Albert Museum, London/Bridgeman Art Library. 72–3, **Frank Kennard**. 74, Dr. Lloyd M. Beidler, Biological Sciences, Florida State University/Science Photo Library. 75, Steve McCutcheon/Frank Lane Picture Agency. 76, Gene Cox/Science Photo Library. 77, M. Voyeux/Gamma/Frank Spooner Pictures. 78, db Photographics, Madison, Connecticut. 79, Leonard Freed/ Magnum/The John Hillelson Agency. 80–1, **Mike Courtney**. 82, Hank Morgan, University of Connecticut/Science Photo Library. 83, Alain Le Garsmeur/Susan Griggs Agency.

Sweet, Sour, Salt, Bitter
84, Constantine Manos/Magnum/The John Hillelson Agency. 87, (top) **Norman Barber**. 88, **Mike Courtney**. 89, **Michael Woods**. 90, (left) Terence Le Goubin/Colorific, (right) Constantine Manos/Magnum/The John Hillelson Agency. 91, Dr. Edward S. Ayensu. 92, Dr. Lloyd M. Beidler, Biological Sciences, Florida State University. 93, Dr. Georg Gerster/The John Hillelson Agency. 94, Carl Purcell/Colorific. 95, Mary Fisher/ Colorific. 96, Richard Kalvar/Magnum/The John Hillelson Agency. 97, *The Oyster Breakfast* by François de Troy. Musée Condé, Chantilly/Bulloz. 98, Guido Mangold/The Image Bank. 99, (both) Kobal Collection. 100, (top) Eddie Adams/Contact/Colorific. (bottom) Christian Vioujard/Gamma/Frank Spooner Pictures. 101, *The Candy Store* (1969) by Richard Estes. Collection of Whitney Museum of American Art. Gift of the Friends of the Whitney Museum of American Art.

The Mechanics of Smell
102, *Christ bearing the Cross* by Hieronymus Bosch. Museum of Fine Arts, Ghent. 104, **Mike Courtney**. 105, (left) Codex Trizulziano, plate 54, folio 30, recto, (right) **Norman Barber**. 106, Wellcome Institute Library, London. 107, **Mike Courtney**. 108–9, **Frank Kennard**. 110, **Norman Barber**. 111, Constantine Manos/Magnum/The John Hillelson Agency. 112, Roland and Sabrina Michaud/ The John Hillelson Agency. 113, Roland and Sabrina Michaud/The John Hillelson Agency. 114, Jean-Paul Ferrero/Ardea Photographics. 115, *An Oleander* by Sir Lawrence Alma-Tadema. Private Collection, USA/Bridgeman Art Library. 116, **Norman Barber**. 117, **Mike Courtney**. 118 (left) Gamma/Frank Spooner

Pictures, (right) Spectrum Colour Library. 119, P. A. Bowman/Natural Science Photos. 120, Mansell Collection. 121, Jacquemart-André Museum, Paris/Gilles Peress/ Magnum/The John Hillelson Agency.

Odor as Communication
122, *Adam and Eve* by Albrecht Durer. British Museum/Fotomas Index. 124, Kobal Collection. 125, **Mike Courtney**. 126 (both) **Norman Barber**. 127, Alexander Lowe/Daily Telegraph Colour Library. 128, Hans Reinhard/Bruce Coleman Limited. 131, BBC Hulton Picture Library.

The Enigma of Smell
132, *Remember Uncle August, The Unhappy Inventor* by George Grosz. © DACS 1984/ Bridgeman Art Library. 134, (bottom), *Le Kid* by Georges Lepape © DACS 1984/Mary Evans Picture Library. 135, Judy Fisher. 136, Whitney Lane/The Image Bank. 137, Marshall Editions Ltd. 138, Wellcome Institute Library, London. 141, Steve Niedorf/The Image Bank. 142, (top) Vloo/Zefa UK Limited, (bottom) **Norman Barber**. 143, Vloo/Zefa UK Limited. 144, *Summer Offering* by Sir Lawrence Alma-Tadema. Private Collection USA/Bridgeman Art Library. 145, BBC Hulton Picture Library.

Scent and Civilized Man
146, Kobal Collection. 148, BBC Hulton Picture Library. 149, (left) Henri Cartier-Bresson/Magnum/The John Hillelson Agency, (right) Mary Evans Picture Library. 150, Mansell Collection. 151, British Museum/Michael Holford. 152, courtesy of Sotheby Parke Bernet. 153, François Guenet/ Gamma/Frank Spooner Pictures. 154, Richard Kalvar/Magnum/The John Hillelson Agency. 157, Victoria and Albert Museum, London/Michael Holford.

Index